CONGESTIVE

HEART FAILURE

IDENTIFYING EARLY SYMPTOMS AND TREATMENT OF HEART FAILURE

Dr. Givens

Bestman

Disclaimer

Copyright © Dr. Givens Bestman 2023. All Rights Reserved.

Contents

INTRODUCTION

Congestive heart failure (CHF) is a serious and potentially life-threatening condition that affects millions of people worldwide. It occurs when the heart is unable to pump blood efficiently, leading to a buildup of fluid in various parts of the body. Recognizing the early symptoms of CHF is crucial for timely intervention and effective management of the condition. In this article, we will explore the early signs and symptoms of CHF and discuss the available treatment options.

Definition of Congestive Heart Failure

Congestive heart failure refers to a condition in which the heart becomes weakened and is unable to pump blood adequately to meet the body's needs. The term "congestive" indicates the accumulation of fluid in the tissues, organs, and body cavities due to the heart's inability to effectively circulate blood.

It is important to note that CHF is not a specific disease but rather a clinical syndrome resulting from various underlying causes, such as coronary artery disease, hypertension, heart valve disorders, and previous heart attacks.

Causes and Risk Factors

Numerous factors can contribute to the development of congestive heart failure. Some of the common causes include:

- Coronary artery disease: Blockages in the blood vessels that supply the heart with oxygen and nutrients can weaken the heart muscle over time.

- High blood pressure: Prolonged hypertension puts extra strain on the heart, leading to its gradual deterioration.

- Cardiomyopathy: Conditions that affect the heart muscle, such as dilated cardiomyopathy or hypertrophic cardiomyopathy, can impair its pumping ability.

- Heart valve disorders: Malfunctioning or damaged heart valves can disrupt the normal flow of blood, causing the heart to work harder.

- Previous heart attacks: Damage to the heart muscle from a heart attack can weaken its ability to pump effectively.

While anyone can develop CHF, certain risk factors increase the likelihood of its occurrence. These include advancing age, obesity, diabetes, smoking, a sedentary lifestyle, a family history of heart disease, and a history of alcohol or drug abuse.

Importance of Early Detection and Treatment

Recognizing the early symptoms of congestive heart failure is crucial for prompt intervention and effective management. Timely diagnosis and treatment can significantly improve the patient's quality of life, slow down the progression of the condition, and reduce the risk of complications. Early intervention can help prevent hospitalizations and emergency room visits, and may even increase life expectancy for individuals living with CHF.

By understanding the signs and symptoms of CHF, individuals and their healthcare providers can work together to initiate appropriate diagnostic evaluations and implement personalized treatment plans. Additionally, lifestyle modifications and adherence to prescribed medications can help individuals manage their symptoms, improve heart function, and enhance overall well-being.

In the following sections of this article, we will delve into the early symptoms of CHF and explore the various diagnostic methods and treatment approaches available.

By gaining a deeper understanding of this condition, we can empower ourselves and others to identify CHF early on and seek timely medical assistance for better outcomes.

Note: It's important to consult a qualified healthcare professional for an accurate diagnosis and personalized treatment plan if you suspect you or someone you know may be experiencing symptoms of congestive heart failure.

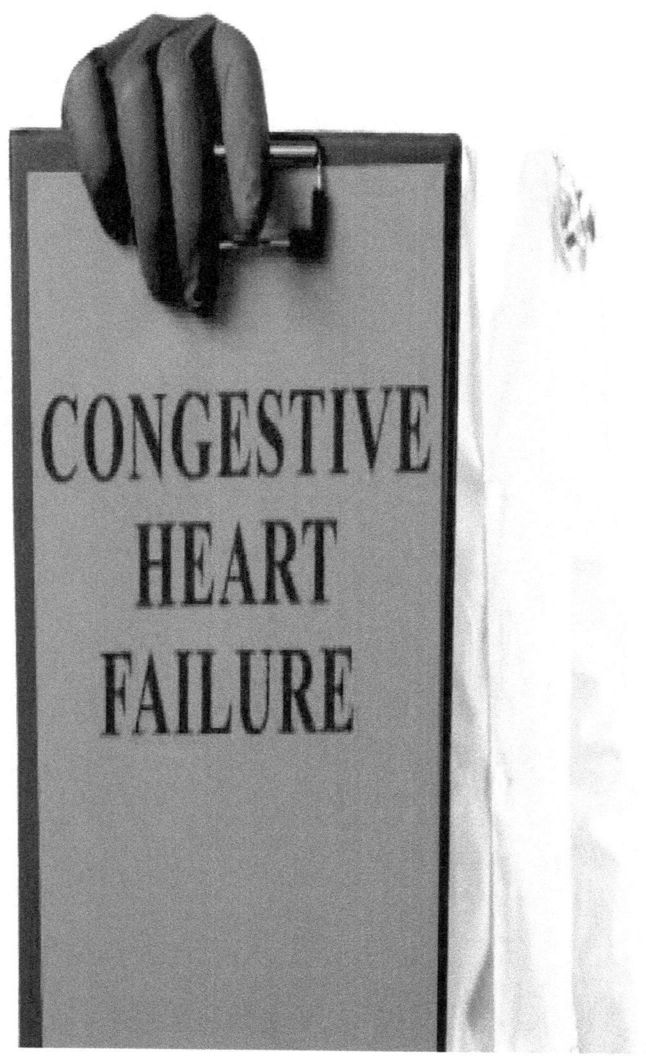

CONGESTIVE
HEART
FAILURE

CHAPTER 1

Understanding the Cardiovascular System

The cardiovascular system, often referred to as the circulatory system, is a complex network of organs, vessels, and cells that serves as the lifeline of the human body. Captivating and detailed, this exploration of the cardiovascular system unravels its intricate workings, highlighting its vital role in sustaining life:

1. The Heart: The Epicenter of Circulation

At the heart of the cardiovascular system lies the heart itself, a remarkable muscular organ about the size of a fist. Acting as a powerful pump, the heart tirelessly propels oxygen-rich blood to all parts of the body and ensures the removal of waste products. Divided into four chambers - the left and right atria and ventricles - the heart orchestrates a synchronized contraction and relaxation process known as the cardiac cycle, which drives the continuous circulation of blood.

2. Arteries: Highways of Vitality

Arteries are thick, muscular blood vessels that carry oxygenated blood away from the heart and deliver it to various organs and tissues throughout the body. These elastic conduits have the crucial task of withstanding the force of the heart's contractions and maintaining a steady flow of blood. As they branch out into smaller vessels called arterioles, arteries ensure that oxygen and nutrients reach every nook and cranny of the body.

3. Veins: The Return Path

In contrast to arteries, veins serve as the return path for blood, carrying deoxygenated blood back to the heart. Veins, aided by one-way valves, navigate through tissues and organs, gradually merging into larger vessels. As they converge, veins transform into two major superhighways: the superior vena cava, which collects blood from the upper body, and the inferior vena cava, responsible for draining blood from the lower body. These two veins unite at the heart's right atrium, preparing for another cycle of circulation.

4. Capillaries: The Microscopic Exchange Points

Capillaries are tiny, delicate vessels that connect arteries and veins at the cellular level. With their vast network, capillaries facilitate the exchange of oxygen, nutrients, and waste products between the bloodstream and surrounding tissues. Through this intricate web of capillaries, oxygen and nutrients diffuse out of the bloodstream to nourish cells, while waste products and carbon dioxide are absorbed and carried away.

5. The Blood: The Vital Fluid

Blood, a remarkable fluid, is the life force coursing through the cardiovascular system. Composed of plasma, red blood cells, white blood cells, and platelets, it performs a multitude of essential functions. Red blood cells transport oxygen, binding it to a molecule called hemoglobin, while white blood cells defend against infections and foreign invaders. Platelets play a crucial role in clotting to prevent excessive bleeding, and plasma carries nutrients, hormones, and waste products throughout the body.

6. Regulation and Control: The Nervous System and Hormones

The cardiovascular system is intricately regulated by both the autonomic nervous system and hormones. The sympathetic and parasympathetic branches of the autonomic nervous system continuously fine-tune heart rate, blood pressure, and vessel constriction, ensuring that blood flow matches the body's needs. Hormones such as adrenaline and noradrenaline, released in response to stress or exercise, also modulate heart rate and blood pressure.

7. Maintenance and Protection: The Role of the Lymphatic System

In addition to the cardiovascular system, the body relies on the lymphatic system to maintain fluid balance, remove waste products, and support immune function. Lymphatic vessels collect excess fluid, known as lymph, from tissues and return it to the bloodstream. The lymphatic system also helps filter and destroy pathogens, contributing to overall cardiovascular health.

Understanding the intricacies of the cardiovascular system is crucial in appreciating its significance and promoting heart health.

By grasping the roles played by the heart, arteries, veins, capillaries, blood, regulation mechanisms, and the lymphatic system, individuals can make informed decisions to support cardiovascular well-being. From adopting a heart-healthy lifestyle to seeking medical care when needed, this understanding empowers individuals to be proactive guardians of their cardiovascular health, ensuring a vibrant and thriving life.

Anatomy and Function of the Heart

The heart, a captivating organ both in its design and its vital function, lies at the core of human existence. Embark on a journey through the intricate anatomy and awe-inspiring functions of the heart, a remarkable powerhouse that keeps life pulsating:

1. The Heart's Structure: A Marvel of Engineering

nestled within the protective confines of the chest cavity, the heart is a complex, muscular organ about the size of a clenched fist.

The four chambers are the right atrium, right ventricle, left atrium, and left ventricle. These chambers are separated by valves that allow blood to flow in one direction, ensuring efficient circulation.

2. Blood Flow: The Engine of Life

The heart's primary function is to pump blood, the life-sustaining fluid, throughout the body. The journey begins with deoxygenated blood entering the heart through the superior and inferior vena cava, into the right atrium. After that, it enters the right ventricle through the tricuspid valve. With a powerful contraction, the right ventricle propels the blood through the pulmonary valve and into the pulmonary artery, leading to the lungs. In the lungs, carbon dioxide is exchanged for oxygen, transforming the blood into its oxygenated state. Oxygen-rich blood then returns to the heart via the pulmonary veins, entering the left atrium.

From there, it flows through the mitral valve into the left ventricle, which contracts forcefully to pump the oxygenated blood through the aortic valve and into the aorta—the body's largest artery.

The blood is then distributed through a vast network of arteries, arterioles, capillaries, venules, and veins, nourishing tissues, and organs before returning to the heart to repeat the cycle.

3. Contraction and Relaxation: The Rhythm of Life

The heart's ability to pump blood depends on a coordinated series of contractions and relaxations. These rhythmic actions are regulated by the electrical system of the heart. The sinoatrial (SA) node, often called the "natural pacemaker," generates electrical impulses that initiate each heartbeat. These impulses travel through specialized conducting pathways, including the atrioventricular (AV) node and the bundle of His, stimulating the contraction of the heart muscle. The synchronized contraction ensures efficient blood ejection, while the subsequent relaxation allows for chambers to refill and prepare for the next cycle.

4. Coronary Circulation: Nourishing the Heart Itself

while the heart tirelessly pumps blood to nourish the body, it also requires its own blood supply.

Coronary arteries, branching off the aorta, supply oxygenated blood to the heart muscle. These vessels meticulously weave through the heart, ensuring that every part receives the nutrients and oxygen it needs to sustain its continuous activity. The coronary veins collect deoxygenated blood and drain it into the right atrium, completing the cycle.

5. Adaptation and Response: Meeting the Body's Demands

The heart possesses an extraordinary ability to adapt and respond to the body's changing needs. During exercise or periods of increased demand, the heart beats faster, increasing the delivery of oxygenated blood to the working muscles. This response is facilitated by the autonomic nervous system, which regulates heart rate and the force of contraction. Hormones, such as adrenaline, also influence the heart's activity, enhancing its performance when necessary.

6. Heart Health: Nurturing the Lifeline

Understanding the anatomy and function of the heart empowers individuals to prioritize their cardiovascular health. By adopting a heart-healthy lifestyle, including regular exercise, a balanced diet, stress management, and avoidance of tobacco products, individuals can support the heart's well-being and reduce the risk of heart disease. Regular check-ups, monitoring blood pressure and cholesterol levels, and seeking medical attention for any concerning symptoms further contribute to maintaining a robust and resilient heart.

In conclusion, the heart's anatomy and function are a testament to the body's remarkable design and its tireless pursuit of sustaining life. From its intricate structure and synchronized contractions to its adaptive nature and vital role in circulation, the heart serves as an awe-inspiring powerhouse. By nurturing the health of this magnificent organ, individuals can cherish the gift of life and enjoy the vibrant rhythm that pulses through their being.

How the Heart Pumps Blood

The heart, an extraordinary marvel of engineering, orchestrates the intricate dance of blood circulation throughout the body. Let's delve into the captivating details of how the heart pumps blood, uncovering the rhythmic symphony that sustains life:

1. A Tale of Four Chambers: The Heart's Inner Sanctum

The heart is divided into four chambers: two atria (the left and right) and two ventricles (also left and right). The receiving chambers are called the atria, and the pumping chambers are called the ventricles. The separation between the chambers is maintained by valves that open and close with precision, ensuring unidirectional blood flow.

2. Atria: Receiving the Baton of Life

Deoxygenated blood, returning from the body's tissues, enters the heart through the superior and inferior vena cava, flowing into the right atrium.

Simultaneously, oxygenated blood from the lungs enters the left atrium through the pulmonary veins.

These atria act as reservoirs, collecting the blood before passing it on to the ventricles.

3. Ventricles: The Powerhouses of the Heart

When the moment arrives, the ventricles spring into action. The right ventricle receives deoxygenated blood from the right atrium by the tricuspid valve. With a robust contraction, it propels the blood through the pulmonary valve, into the pulmonary artery, and toward the lungs. In the lungs, carbon dioxide is exchanged for oxygen, transforming the blood into its oxygenated state.

Meanwhile, the left ventricle receives oxygenated blood from the left atrium through the mitral valve. It contracts forcefully, generating the power required to propel the oxygenated blood through the aortic valve and into the aorta—the body's largest artery. From there, the blood embarks on a grand journey, flowing through arteries, arterioles, and capillaries, nourishing every cell and tissue it encounters.

4. The Role of Valves: Guardians of Unidirectional Flow

Valves play a crucial role in the heart's pumping action by ensuring the flow of blood is unidirectional. The tricuspid valve, located between the right atrium and right ventricle, and the mitral valve, situated between the left atrium and left ventricle, prevent backflow of blood during ventricular contractions.

Similarly, the pulmonary valve guards the exit of the right ventricle, preventing blood from flowing back into the ventricle after it is pumped into the pulmonary artery. The aortic valve, located at the exit of the left ventricle, performs a similar duty, ensuring blood flows forward into the aorta without regurgitation.

5. The Synchronized Dance: Contraction and Relaxation

The heart's pumping action follows a synchronized dance of contraction and relaxation. The contraction, known as systole, is initiated by electrical impulses generated by the sinoatrial (SA) node—the natural pacemaker of the heart.

These impulses spread through specialized conducting pathways, stimulating the atria to contract, forcing blood into the ventricles.

After a brief pause, the atrioventricular (AV) node relays the electrical signal to the ventricles, causing them to contract forcefully. This propels blood into the pulmonary artery and aorta, initiating circulation. Following the contraction, a period of relaxation, known as diastole, allows the ventricles to refill with blood, preparing for the next cycle.

6. The Pulse of Life: Feeling the Heartbeat

The rhythmic pumping action of the heart creates a tangible sensation—the pulse. As blood is propelled from the heart, it creates a surge of pressure that can be felt in arteries throughout the body. Monitoring the pulse provides valuable information about heart rate and rhythm, offering insights into cardiovascular health.

7. Maintaining the Rhythm: Regulatory Mechanisms

The heart's pumping action is regulated by the autonomic nervous system and influenced by hormones. The sympathetic nervous system accelerates heart rate and increases the force of contractions, preparing the body for action or stress. In contrast, the parasympathetic nervous system slows the heart rate and promotes relaxation.

Hormones, such as adrenaline, released in response to stress or physical exertion, also influence heart rate and the strength of contractions, ensuring the heart responds appropriately to the body's needs.

Understanding how the heart pumps blood unveils the intricate symphony that sustains life. From the coordinated actions of the atria and ventricles to the guardianship of valves, every component plays a vital role. The heart's rhythmic pulsations remind us of the wondrous symphony within, a testament to our existence and a constant reminder of the vibrant, life-giving force that resides within us all.

The Role of the Circulatory System

The circulatory system, a captivating and intricate network, serves as the life-enabling highway within the human body. Prepare to embark on a captivating journey as we unveil the remarkable role this system plays in sustaining life:

1. Oxygen and Nutrient Delivery: Nourishing Every Cell

At the heart of the circulatory system's mission lies the vital task of delivering oxygen and nutrients to every cell and tissue in the body. Oxygen, obtained through respiration, enters the bloodstream in the lungs and binds to red blood cells, forming a vital partnership. These oxygen-rich red blood cells journey through arteries, arterioles, and capillaries, where they release oxygen to nourish cells and tissues. Simultaneously, nutrients derived from the digestion of food are absorbed into the bloodstream, further fueling the body's needs.

2. Waste Removal: Cleansing the Body's Pathways

As oxygen and nutrients are delivered, the circulatory system also serves as a vital waste removal system. Waste products, such as carbon dioxide and metabolic byproducts, are picked up by the blood as it passes through capillaries. This waste-laden blood is then transported through venules and veins back to the heart and eventually to the lungs and kidneys, where these waste products are eliminated from the body. The circulatory system's efficient waste removal mechanisms ensure the body's metabolic balance and overall health.

3. Immune Defense: Safeguarding Against Invaders

The circulatory system plays a crucial role in the body's immune defense. White blood cells, the soldiers of the immune system, are transported through the bloodstream to detect and neutralize harmful pathogens, such as bacteria, viruses, and other foreign invaders. These vigilant defenders patrol the body, ensuring that infectious agents are identified and eradicated, helping to maintain overall health and well-being.

4. Temperature Regulation: Balancing the Body's Climate

The circulatory system contributes to the body's temperature regulation. As blood circulates, it carries heat throughout the body, helping to maintain a stable internal temperature. When the body is too warm, blood vessels near the skin's surface dilate, allowing excess heat to escape through the process of sweating. Conversely, when the body is cold, blood vessels constrict to minimize heat loss, ensuring essential warmth is conserved in vital organs.

5. Hormone Transport: Facilitating Communication

within Hormones, chemical messengers produced by various glands, play a vital role in regulating bodily functions. The circulatory system acts as a carrier for these hormones, allowing them to travel to their target organs and tissues. Through the bloodstream, hormones communicate instructions, coordinating essential processes such as growth, metabolism, reproduction, and mood regulation.

6. Blood Clotting: Repairing and Protecting

In the event of injury, the circulatory system orchestrates the remarkable process of blood clotting. Platelets, small cell fragments, and clotting factors in the blood work together to form a clot, sealing off the injured blood vessel and preventing excessive bleeding. This vital mechanism repairs damaged vessels, protects against blood loss, and initiates the healing process.

7. Adaptation to Body's Needs: Dynamic and Responsive

One of the circulatory system's most captivating qualities is its ability to adapt to the body's changing needs. During physical activity or exercise, the heart pumps faster, and blood vessels dilate, ensuring increased oxygen and nutrient delivery to working muscles. Conversely, during rest, the system slows down, conserving energy and maintaining a steady flow to support essential functions.

The role of the circulatory system is captivating and essential to sustaining life. From oxygen and nutrient delivery to waste removal, immune defense, temperature regulation, hormone transport, blood clotting, and adaptation to the body's needs, this intricate network ensures the body functions harmoniously. By appreciating the remarkable role of the circulatory system, we gain a deeper understanding of the delicate balance that allows us to thrive and experience the wonders of life.

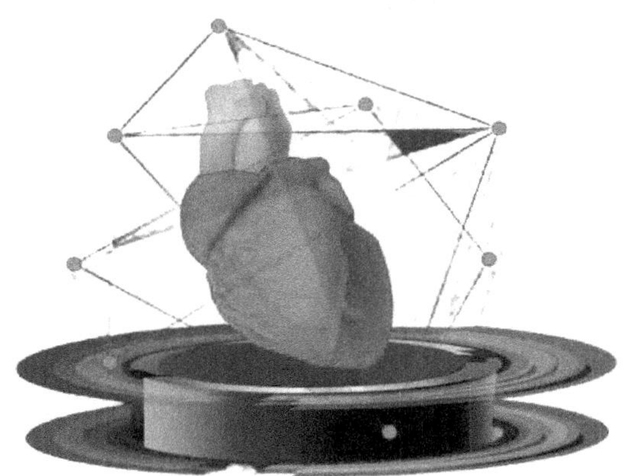

CHAPTER 2

Early Symptoms of Congestive Heart Failure: Recognizing the Warning Signs

Congestive heart failure (CHF) is a delicate condition that needs immediate medical attention. Identifying the early symptoms of CHF is crucial for timely diagnosis and intervention, potentially improving outcomes and quality of life. Let's explore the professional, captivating, and detailed list of early symptoms to watch out for:

1. Fatigue and Reduced Stamina:

One of the earliest signs of CHF is an unexplained and persistent fatigue. Individuals may feel unusually tired, even after minimal physical exertion or daily activities. Simple tasks that were once effortless may now leave them feeling exhausted and lacking stamina.

2. Shortness of Breath:

Another common early symptom is shortness of breath or dyspnea. Individuals may find it increasingly difficult to catch their breath, especially during physical activity or when lying flat. They may experience a sensation of breathlessness or a need to take frequent shallow breaths. In some cases, this symptom may even manifest during rest.

3. Fluid Retention and Swelling:

Fluid retention, known as edema, is a classic early symptom of CHF. It commonly manifests as swelling in the feet, ankles, legs, or abdomen. The swelling may be more noticeable at the end of the day or after prolonged periods of sitting or standing. Individuals may also experience sudden weight gain due to fluid accumulation.

4. Persistent Cough:

A chronic and persistent cough can be an early indication of CHF. This cough may be dry or accompanied by white or pink-tinged phlegm. It often worsens at night or when lying flat due to fluid accumulation in the lungs.

5. Rapid or Irregular Heartbeat:

Heart palpitations, characterized by a rapid or irregular heartbeat, may occur in the early stages of CHF. Individuals may feel their heart beating or fluttering in their chest. This symptom may be accompanied by a sense of anxiety or discomfort.

6. Reduced Appetite and Nausea:

Early symptoms of CHF can also manifest as a decreased appetite and feelings of nausea. Individuals may experience a loss of interest in food or feel full quickly even after consuming small meals. Nausea may be persistent or occur intermittently.

7. Difficulty Sleeping:

Sleep disturbances can be an early warning sign of CHF. Individuals may find it challenging to fall asleep or stay asleep due to symptoms such as shortness of breath, coughing, or discomfort. They may wake up feeling restless or unrefreshed.

8. Cognitive Changes:

In some cases, early symptoms of CHF may include cognitive changes such as confusion, difficulty concentrating, or memory problems. These changes may be subtle initially but can progress over time if left untreated.

It's important to note that these early symptoms can be nonspecific and may overlap with other health conditions. However, if you experience any of these symptoms persistently or if they worsen over time, it's crucial to seek medical evaluation. Early detection of CHF allows for timely intervention, potentially preventing further damage to the heart and improving prognosis.

Remember, the presence of these early symptoms does not provide a definitive diagnosis of CHF. Only a qualified healthcare professional can assess your symptoms, perform diagnostic tests, and provide an accurate diagnosis. If you or a loved one experiences any concerning symptoms, don't delay—seek medical attention promptly to ensure the best possible care and management of your cardiovascular health.

General Symptoms and Signs

Congestive heart failure (CHF) is a complex condition that affects millions of people worldwide. Recognizing the general signs and symptoms of CHF is essential for early detection, prompt medical intervention, and improved management of this serious condition. Let's explore the professional, captivating, and detailed list of general signs and symptoms associated with CHF:

1. Shortness of Breath (Dyspnea):

One of the hallmark symptoms of CHF is shortness of breath. Individuals may experience difficulty breathing, especially during physical activity or when lying flat. The sensation of breathlessness may be accompanied by rapid breathing or a feeling of suffocation. Some individuals may need to prop themselves up with extra pillows to alleviate this symptom.

2. Fatigue and Weakness:

Fatigue and generalized weakness are common symptoms of CHF. Individuals may feel unusually tired and lacking in energy, even after performing simple tasks or activities that were previously effortless. This persistent fatigue can significantly impact daily functioning and quality of life.

3. Swelling and Edema:

Fluid retention and swelling medically referred to as edema, often occur in CHF. Swelling typically affects the legs, ankles, feet, and sometimes the abdomen. The swelling may worsen during the day, especially after prolonged periods of sitting or standing. Individuals may notice a sudden increase in weight due to fluid accumulation.

4. Persistent Cough:

A persistent, dry cough is a frequently reported symptom of CHF. The cough may be worse at night or when lying flat and may be accompanied by the production of white or pink-tinged phlegm. It occurs due to fluid accumulation in the lungs, irritating the airways and triggering coughing.

5. Rapid or Irregular Heartbeat:

Heart palpitations, characterized by a rapid or irregular heartbeat, may occur in CHF. Individuals may feel their heart racing, fluttering, or pounding in their chest. This symptom can be alarming and may be accompanied by dizziness or a sense of anxiety.

6. Reduced Exercise Tolerance:

Individuals with CHF often experience a decline in exercise tolerance. Activities that were once manageable may become increasingly difficult and exhausting. They may need to take frequent breaks or rest more frequently during physical exertion.

7. Swollen Veins in the Neck:

Engorged neck veins can be a telltale sign of CHF. These veins may appear distended, prominent, or swollen when individuals are in an upright position. This occurs due to increased pressure in the veins returning blood to the heart.

8. Poor Appetite and Nausea:

CHF can lead to a decreased appetite and feelings of nausea. Individuals may have a reduced interest in food, experience early satiety, or feel nauseated. These symptoms can contribute to unintended weight loss and malnutrition if not addressed.

9. Difficulty Sleeping and Restlessness:

Sleep disturbances are common in CHF. Individuals may have difficulty falling asleep or staying asleep due to shortness of breath, coughing, or discomfort. They may awaken frequently during the night, feel restless, or have vivid dreams. This lack of restful sleep can further contribute to fatigue and overall fatigue.

10. Mental Confusion and Impaired Thinking:

In advanced stages of CHF, individuals may experience mental confusion, difficulty concentrating, or memory problems. This can be attributed to reduced blood flow and oxygen supply to the brain, impacting cognitive function.

It's important to note that these general signs and symptoms of CHF can vary in severity and may overlap with other health conditions. If you or a loved one experience any of these symptoms, it's crucial to seek medical evaluation for an accurate diagnosis and appropriate management.

Remember, early detection and intervention can greatly improve results and quality of life for individuals with CHF. If you notice any concerning signs or symptoms, don't delay—consult a healthcare professional promptly to ensure timely and comprehensive care.

Fatigue and Weakness

Fatigue and weakness are common companions for individuals living with congestive heart failure (CHF). These debilitating symptoms can significantly impact their daily lives and overall well-being. In this exploration, we delve into the professional, captivating, and detailed understanding of fatigue and weakness in CHF patients.

1. Overwhelming Exhaustion:

Fatigue in CHF goes beyond normal tiredness—it is an overwhelming exhaustion that persists even after ample rest. Individuals may wake up feeling tired and lack the energy to perform routine activities. Simple tasks that were once effortless become arduous challenges. This persistent weariness saps their motivation and leaves them longing for relief.

2. Physical and Mental Drain:

Fatigue and weakness affect both the body and the mind. Physical tasks that require strength and endurance become increasingly difficult. Climbing stairs, carrying groceries, or even getting dressed can be exhausting endeavors. Alongside the physical fatigue, individuals may experience mental fatigue, leading to difficulty concentrating, memory lapses, and reduced cognitive function.

3. Impact on Daily Activities:

The impact of fatigue and weakness on daily activities cannot be overstated. CHF patients often find themselves limited in what they can accomplish.

Activities they once enjoyed may be postponed or abandoned altogether. Their energy reserves are depleted quickly, leaving little room for participation in social events, hobbies, or quality time with loved ones. The burden of fatigue casts a shadow over their lives.

4. Underlying Mechanisms:

Fatigue and weakness in CHF result from a combination of factors. The heart's impaired pumping ability leads to reduced blood flow and oxygen delivery to the body's tissues and organs. As a result, muscles receive insufficient oxygen and nutrients, contributing to fatigue. Additionally, fluid retention and the accumulation of metabolic waste products further contribute to feelings of weakness and exhaustion.

5. Interplay with Other Symptoms:

Fatigue and weakness often coexist with other symptoms of CHF, such as shortness of breath and swelling. The combination of these symptoms can create a vicious cycle.

For instance, shortness of breath during physical exertion can limit activity levels, leading to deconditioning and increased fatigue. This interplay underscores the importance of comprehensive management strategies.

6. Psychological Toll:

The burden of fatigue and weakness extends beyond the physical realm, impacting individuals psychologically. Chronic fatigue can lead to feelings of frustration, irritability, and a sense of helplessness. The inability to engage in activities that once brought joy can result in sadness and depression. Supportive care addressing the emotional well-being of CHF patients is crucial in managing the overall impact of these symptoms.

7. Managing Fatigue and Weakness:

Addressing fatigue and weakness in CHF involves a multifaceted approach. Healthcare professionals work closely with patients to develop personalized strategies.

This may include optimizing medication regimens, incorporating regular physical activity and exercise, providing dietary guidance, managing comorbidities, and ensuring adequate rest and sleep.

A holistic approach to symptom management can help alleviate fatigue and improve overall quality of life.

8. Seeking Support:

If you or a loved one experiences persistent fatigue and weakness, it is crucial to seek medical support. Healthcare professionals can assess the underlying causes, evaluate the effectiveness of current treatments, and provide recommendations for tailored interventions. Additionally, support from family, friends, and support groups can offer emotional support and practical assistance in managing the challenges posed by these symptoms.

Fatigue and weakness in CHF patients are not simply fleeting moments of tiredness—they are enduring companions that impact every aspect of their lives.

By recognizing the profound burden these symptoms carry and implementing comprehensive strategies for management, we can empower individuals living with CHF to regain control, improve their energy levels, and enhance their overall well-being.

Shortness of Breath

Shortness of breath, medically known as dyspnea, is a hallmark symptom of congestive heart failure (CHF). It is a complex and distressing sensation that deserves our attention. In this professional, captivating, and detailed exploration, we will uncover the significance of shortness of breath in CHF and its impact on individuals' lives.

1. The Hidden Struggle:

Shortness of breath is a relentless foe that plagues those with CHF. It manifests as a feeling of breathlessness, as if the very air they depend on has become scarce.

Simple activities that were once effortless, such as walking up a flight of stairs or even engaging in light conversation, can trigger a suffocating sensation. This hidden struggle leaves individuals grappling for air and yearning for relief.

2. Mechanisms at Play:

In CHF, shortness of breath arises from the impaired pumping ability of the heart. As the heart weakens, it struggles to effectively circulate blood throughout the body, resulting in a backup of fluid in the lungs. This accumulation of fluid in the pulmonary system leads to increased pressure and compromises the exchange of oxygen and carbon dioxide. The body's vital oxygen supply becomes limited, and the individual experiences the distressing sensation of breathlessness.

3. Onset and Progression:

Shortness of breath in CHF often starts gradually and worsens over time. Initially, it may only occur during strenuous activities or exertion. However, as the condition advances, it can occur with minimal exertion or even at rest. Individuals may find it challenging to lie flat and may need to prop themselves up with extra pillows to alleviate the sensation of suffocation.

4. Impact on Daily Life:

The impact of shortness of breath on individuals with CHF cannot be understated. It permeates every aspect of their lives, hindering their ability to perform routine tasks and participate in activities they once enjoyed. Simple activities like getting dressed, showering, or preparing meals become arduous challenges. The constant struggle for breath can lead to feelings of frustration, anxiety, and a sense of confinement.

5. Psychological Burden:

Shortness of breath in CHF carries a significant psychological burden. The fear of not being able to breathe adequately engenders anxiety and can contribute to a diminished quality of life. Individuals may limit their physical activities and social interactions due to the distressing symptoms, leading to social isolation and a loss of independence.

6. Diagnostic Significance:

The presence and severity of shortness of breath in CHF are vital diagnostic indicators.

Healthcare professionals carefully assess the onset, duration, and response to specific interventions to help guide treatment decisions. Monitoring changes in shortness of breath can provide valuable insights into disease progression and response to therapy.

7. Management and Support:

Addressing shortness of breath in CHF requires a multidimensional approach. Healthcare professionals employ various strategies, including medication adjustments, lifestyle modifications, and pulmonary rehabilitation programs, to alleviate this distressing symptom. In addition, emotional support, education, and self-care strategies play a crucial role in helping individuals manage their symptoms and improve their overall well-being.

8. Seeking Medical Attention:

If you or a loved one experiences persistent or worsening shortness of breathe, it is essential to seek immediate medical attention.

Prompt evaluation by a healthcare professional can help determine the underlying cause, whether related to CHF or another condition, and guide appropriate interventions.

Shortness of breath in CHF is not merely a physical sensation—it is a profound and challenging experience that demands our attention. By understanding its mechanisms, impact, and the importance of timely intervention, we can offer support and compassion to those grappling with this invisible struggle. Together, let us shed light on the hidden burdens of shortness of breath in congestive heart failure and strive for improved care and quality of life.

Swelling and Edema

Swelling and edema, often observed in individuals with congestive heart failure (CHF), paint a vivid picture of the intricate challenges faced by these patients.

This professional, captivating, and detailed exploration delves into the significance of swelling and edema, unraveling the puzzle of fluid retention in CHF patients.

1. The Visible Manifestation:

Swelling, commonly referred to as edema, is the accumulation of fluid in the body's tissues. In CHF, it most commonly occurs in the legs, ankles, and feet, but can also affect other areas such as the abdomen and hands. This visible manifestation of fluid retention is a tangible reminder of the underlying cardiovascular imbalance.

2. Mechanisms at Play:

In CHF, the heart's weakened pumping ability causes inadequate blood circulation. As a result, fluid can back up in the veins, leading to increased pressure in the capillaries. This pressure forces fluid out of the blood vessels and into the surrounding tissues, resulting in swelling and edema. The fluid retention puzzle is an intricate interplay of impaired cardiac function and the body's compensatory mechanisms.

3. Progression and Severity:

Swelling and edema in CHF patients may start gradually, initially appearing in the feet or ankles, especially after prolonged periods of standing or sitting.

Over time, the swelling can worsen and spread to other parts of the body, becoming more persistent and pronounced. It is essential to monitor and assess the severity of edema as it can provide insights into the progression of CHF and the effectiveness of treatment interventions.

4. Impact on Daily Life:

The impact of swelling and edema reaches far beyond physical discomfort. The visible swelling can affect body image and self-esteem, leading to feelings of self-consciousness and embarrassment.

The swollen limbs may become heavy and cumbersome, making it challenging to move and engage in normal activities. Putting on shoes or clothing can become a struggle, further adding to the frustration and limitations experienced by CHF patients.

5. Signs of Fluid Overload:

Swelling and edema serve as important indicators of fluid overload in CHF.

Other signs of fluid accumulation may include rapid weight gain, bloating, and distention of the abdomen. These signs should not be ignored, as they may indicate worsening heart failure and the need for medical intervention.

6. Diuretic Therapy:

Managing swelling and edema often involves the use of diuretic medications. These medications help increase urine production, facilitating the removal of excess fluid from the body. Healthcare professionals carefully assess the appropriate dosage and timing of diuretics to strike a balance between reducing fluid retention and maintaining electrolyte balance.

7. Lifestyle Modifications:

In addition to medications, lifestyle modifications play a crucial role in managing swelling and edema. This may include dietary changes, such as reducing sodium intake, as excessive salt can contribute to fluid retention. Regular physical activity, when appropriate, can also help improve circulation and reduce fluid buildup.

8. Monitoring and Reporting:

Individuals with CHF should closely monitor swelling and edema and report any changes to their healthcare providers. Tracking the extent of swelling, documenting weight fluctuations, and reporting symptoms of fluid overload are essential for healthcare professionals to evaluate the effectiveness of treatment and make necessary adjustments.

9. Elevating the Limbs:

To alleviate swelling and edema, elevating the affected limbs above the level of the heart can help promote fluid drainage and reduce swelling. This simple yet effective strategy can provide temporary relief and aid in the management of fluid retention.

10. Importance of Compliance:

Managing swelling and edema in CHF requires consistent adherence to treatment plans. It is vital for individuals to take prescribed medications as directed, follow recommended dietary guidelines, and maintain regular follow-up appointments with their healthcare providers.

Compliance with these measures is crucial for effectively managing fluid retention and promoting overall heart health.

Swelling and edema in CHF patients are not merely superficial manifestations—they are physical reminders of the complex imbalances within the cardiovascular system. By understanding the mechanisms, impact, and management strategies associated with fluid retention, we can work towards improving the lives of CHF patients, reducing their discomfort, and restoring a sense of normalcy.

Rapid or Irregular Heartbeat

A rapid or irregular heartbeat is a common occurrence in individuals living with congestive heart failure (CHF). It serves as a poignant reminder of the challenges faced by these patients and warrants our attention.

In this captivating and detailed exploration, we delve into the significance of rapid or irregular heartbeat in CHF patients, unveiling the rhythm of the struggling heart.

1. The Symphony of the Heart:

The heartbeat, a symphony of electrical impulses and muscle contractions, is the life force that keeps our bodies functioning. In CHF, this symphony becomes disrupted, leading to alterations in heart rhythm. A rapid or irregular heartbeat, also known as arrhythmia, can occur as the heart struggles to maintain its normal rhythm and balance.

2. Mechanisms at Play:

CHF can cause electrical abnormalities within the heart, resulting in arrhythmias.

The weakened heart muscles and compromised blood flow can disrupt the electrical signals that coordinate the heart's contractions. This can lead to rapid, irregular, or skipped beats. Additionally, certain medications used to manage CHF can also influence heart rhythm.

3. Signs and Symptoms:

Rapid or irregular heartbeat in CHF patients may present with palpitations, a sensation of fluttering, pounding, or racing in the chest. Individuals may be acutely aware of their heartbeats, which can cause anxiety and distress. Other accompanying symptoms may include dizziness,

lighteadedness, shortness of breath, and fatigue. The onset
and severity of these symptoms can vary among individuals.

4. Impact on Daily Life:

The presence of a rapid or irregular heartbeat can
significantly impact the daily lives of CHF patients. The
unpredictable nature of arrhythmias can be unsettling and
may lead to a heightened sense of anxiety. Individuals may
feel limited in their activities, fearful of triggering or
exacerbating their symptoms. The impact extends beyond
physical limitations and can influence emotional well-being,
social interactions, and overall quality of life.

5. Types of Arrhythmias:

Various types of arrhythmias can occur in CHF, including
atrial fibrillation (AFib), ventricular tachycardia (VT), and
premature ventricular contractions (PVCs). Each has its
unique characteristics and implications for patient
management.

It is important for healthcare professionals to accurately
diagnose and classify the specific arrhythmia to guide
appropriate treatment strategies.

6. Treatment Approaches:

Managing rapid or irregular heartbeat in CHF involves a multifaceted approach. Healthcare professionals may prescribe medications to regulate heart rhythm and control the heart rate. In some cases, interventions such as cardioversion, catheter ablation, or implantable devices like pacemakers or defibrillators may be recommended to restore and maintain a normal heart rhythm.

Lifestyle modifications, such as reducing stress, avoiding triggers, and adhering to medication regimens, also play a crucial role in arrhythmia management.

7. Monitoring and Follow-up:

Regular monitoring and follow-up with healthcare providers are essential for individuals with CHF and arrhythmias. This allows for close observation of heart rhythm patterns, evaluation of medication effectiveness, and adjustment of treatment plans as needed.

Timely reporting of any new or worsening symptoms is crucial to ensure comprehensive and individualized care.

8. Addressing Underlying Causes:

While managing the symptoms of rapid or irregular heartbeat is important, addressing the underlying causes is equally essential. Optimal management of CHF, including medication adherence, lifestyle modifications, and timely interventions, can help alleviate the burden on the heart and improve overall cardiac function. By addressing the root cause, healthcare professionals strive to create a more stable and harmonious rhythm within the heart.

Rapid or irregular heartbeat in CHF patients is not a mere irregularity—it is a reminder of the intricate dance between the heart's electrical impulses and its struggle to maintain balance. By understanding the mechanisms, impact, and management strategies associated with arrhythmias, we can empower CHF patients to navigate the rhythm of their lives with greater confidence, improved well-being, and enhanced cardiac health.

CHAPTER 3

Diagnosis and Evaluation of Congestive Heart Failure

Diagnosing and evaluating congestive heart failure (CHF) requires a comprehensive and systematic approach to unravel the complexities of this condition. In this comprehensive and detailed exploration, we delve into the significance of diagnosis and evaluation in CHF, guiding healthcare professionals in their quest for clarity and optimal patient care.

1. Patient History and Physical Examination:

The journey towards diagnosing CHF begins with a thorough patient history and physical examination. Healthcare professionals carefully listen to the patient's symptoms, medical history, and family history, paying particular attention to signs and symptoms such as shortness of breath, fatigue, swelling, and exercise intolerance.

A comprehensive physical examination provides valuable insights into the patient's cardiovascular status, including the assessment of heart sounds, presence of murmurs, elevated jugular venous pressure, and signs of fluid retention.

2. Diagnostic Tests:

A range of diagnostic tests aids in the evaluation of CHF, helping to confirm the diagnosis, assess its severity, identify underlying causes, and guide appropriate management strategies. These tests may include:

- **Electrocardiogram (ECG):** This non-invasive test records the electrical activity of the heart, identifying abnormalities in heart rhythm and detecting signs of myocardial damage or enlargement.

- **Echocardiography:** This imaging test utilizes sound waves to create detailed images of the heart's structure, size, and function.

It assesses parameters such as ejection fraction (EF), ventricular dimensions, valvular abnormalities, and estimates of pulmonary artery pressure.

- **Chest X-ray:** This imaging technique provides valuable information about the heart's size, shape, and position. It helps identify signs of fluid accumulation in the lungs and pleural effusions.

- **Cardiac MRI:** Magnetic resonance imaging (MRI) provides detailed images of the heart's structure and function. It can assess ventricular volumes, regional wall motion abnormalities, and identify areas of myocardial scarring.

- **Cardiac CT Scan:** Computed tomography (CT) scans can provide three-dimensional images of the heart, aiding in the evaluation of coronary artery disease and identifying structural abnormalities.

- **Blood Tests:** Blood tests measure various biomarkers such as brain natriuretic peptide (BNP) or N-terminal pro-BNP (NT-proBNP), which can help assess cardiac stress and determine the severity of heart failure.

- **Exercise Stress Test:** This test evaluates the heart's response to physical exertion, measuring parameters such as heart rate, blood pressure, and symptoms during exercise. It helps assess exercise capacity and reveals any underlying limitations.

- **Coronary Angiography:** In some cases, coronary angiography may be performed to assess the presence of coronary artery disease, which can contribute to CHF.

3. Classification and Staging:

Once the diagnosis of CHF is confirmed, healthcare professionals classify and stage the condition, aiding in treatment planning and prognostication.

The New York Heart Association (NYHA) functional classification system categorizes patients into classes based on the severity of their symptoms and limitations. The

American College of Cardiology/American Heart Association (ACC/AHA) staging system evaluates the progression of the disease, considering factors such as structural heart disease, symptoms, and hospitalizations.

4. Assessment of Underlying Causes and Comorbidities:

Identifying the underlying causes of CHF and assessing comorbidities is crucial for comprehensive management. This may involve further investigations such as coronary angiography, thyroid function tests, pulmonary function tests, and sleep studies, depending on clinical suspicion and patient-specific factors. Evaluating comorbid conditions such as hypertension, diabetes, kidney disease, and valvular heart disease provides a holistic understanding of the patient's cardiovascular health and guides targeted interventions.

5. Multidisciplinary Collaboration:

The diagnosis and evaluation of CHF often require a multidisciplinary approach, involving collaboration between cardiologists, primary care physicians, nurses, imaging specialists, and other healthcare professionals. This collaborative effort ensures a comprehensive assessment, accurate diagnosis, and personalized treatment plans tailored to the unique needs of each patient.

6. Ongoing Monitoring and Follow-up:

CHF is a dynamic condition that requires ongoing monitoring and follow-up. Regular assessment of symptoms, physical examination findings, and objective measures such as echocardiography and biomarker levels helps gauge treatment response, disease progression, and the need for adjustments in therapy. Close communication with patients and their caregivers is vital to ensure adherence to treatment plans, address concerns, and optimize long-term outcomes.

The diagnosis and evaluation of CHF involve a meticulous process that combines clinical expertise, advanced diagnostic tests, and collaboration among healthcare professionals. By unraveling the complexities of this condition, we empower healthcare providers to embark on a path towards clarity, enabling timely interventions, tailored management strategies, and improved patient outcomes.

Medical History and Physical Examination

Thoroughly assessing the medical history and conducting a comprehensive physical examination are fundamental steps in diagnosing and managing congestive heart failure (CHF). This comprehensive and detailed exploration delves into the significance of medical history and physical examination, highlighting the valuable clues they provide to unravel the complexities of CHF and guide optimal patient care.

1. Medical History Assessment:

Obtaining a detailed medical history is the cornerstone of evaluating a patient with suspected or known CHF.

Healthcare professionals engage in a comprehensive dialogue with the patient, covering the following aspects:

- **Symptoms:** Inquiring about symptoms such as shortness of breath, fatigue, exercise intolerance, orthopnea (difficulty breathing while lying flat), paroxysmal nocturnal dyspnea (awakening with breathlessness at night), cough, chest pain, palpitations, and swelling in the legs or abdomen. Understanding the onset, duration, and progression of these symptoms provides critical insights into the patient's clinical presentation.

- **Past Medical History:** Exploring the presence of pre-existing conditions that can contribute to the development or worsening of CHF, such as hypertension, coronary artery disease, valvular heart disease, diabetes mellitus, obesity, chronic kidney disease, and previous myocardial infarction. Identifying previous cardiac interventions, such as angioplasty, coronary artery bypass grafting (CABG), or valve replacement, is also essential.

- **Medications:** Reviewing the patient's medication list, including current prescriptions, over-the-counter medications, and herbal supplements. Paying attention to medications that can impact cardiac function, such as beta-blockers, angiotensin-converting enzyme (ACE) inhibitors, angiotensin receptor blockers (ARBs), diuretics, and antiarrhythmic drugs.

- **Family History:** Exploring the presence of cardiovascular diseases in the patient's immediate family, as certain conditions can have a genetic predisposition.

- **Lifestyle Factors:** Inquiring about lifestyle factors that can contribute to the development or exacerbation of CHF, such as smoking, excessive alcohol consumption, sedentary lifestyle, and dietary habits.

- **Social History:** Understanding the patient's living situation, support system, occupation, and potential exposures to toxins or substances that can affect cardiac health.

2. Comprehensive Physical Examination:

Performing a systematic and detailed physical examination is crucial in evaluating a patient with suspected CHF. The examination aims to assess the cardiovascular system and detect signs of fluid overload and cardiac dysfunction. Key components of the physical examination include:

- **Vital Signs:** Measuring the patient's blood pressure, heart rate, respiratory rate, and temperature.
  These basic vital signs provide important baseline information for ongoing monitoring and help assess the hemodynamic stability of the patient.

- **General Appearance:** Observing the patient's overall appearance, noting any signs of respiratory distress, cyanosis (bluish discoloration of the lips or extremities), or peripheral edema. Evaluating the patient's overall nutritional status and assessing for cachexia (severe muscle wasting) or obesity, which can have implications for CHF management.

- **Jugular Venous Pressure (JVP):** Assessing the jugular venous pulsation and estimating the JVP, which reflects the central venous pressure. Elevated JVP is suggestive of fluid overload and right-sided heart dysfunction, common in CHF.

- **Heart Auscultation:** Carefully listening to the heart sounds using a stethoscope.

Identifying abnormal heart sounds, such as murmurs, gallops (additional heart sounds), or rubs, can provide insights into cardiac structure and function. Characterizing the presence, timing, and intensity of these sounds is crucial for appropriate diagnosis and further evaluation.

- **Pulmonary Examination:** Listening to the lung fields for the presence of crackles, wheezes, or decreased breath sounds. These findings can indicate the presence of pulmonary congestion or underlying lung pathology.

- **Peripheral Edema:** Assessing for peripheral edema, particularly in the lower extremities, which can indicate fluid retention associated with CHF. Examining for pitting edema by applying pressure to the affected area can help assess its severity.

- **Abdominal Examination:** Palpating the abdomen for hepatomegaly (enlarged liver), which can be a sign of right-sided heart failure.
Assessing for ascites (fluid accumulation in the abdominal cavity) may also be indicative of advanced CHF.

- **Extremity Examination:** Examining the extremities for signs of peripheral arterial disease, such as diminished pulses, cool skin, or trophic changes (skin or nail abnormalities). Assessing for the presence of peripheral edema, varicose veins, or ulcers is important to evaluate the circulatory status and assess the impact of CHF on the peripheral vascular system.

The medical history assessment and physical examination serve as crucial initial steps in diagnosing and evaluating CHF. They provide valuable clues that guide further investigations, help determine the severity and underlying etiology of CHF, and facilitate personalized treatment plans. By unraveling the intricate web of patient history and physical findings, healthcare professionals pave the way toward optimal management and improved outcomes for individuals with CHF.

Diagnostic Tests and Procedures

Diagnosing and evaluating congestive heart failure (CHF) requires a comprehensive array of diagnostic tests and procedures to gather valuable insights into cardiac structure, function, and underlying causes. In this comprehensive and detailed exploration, we delve into the significance of diagnostic tests and procedures in CHF, shedding light on their role in achieving accurate assessment and guiding optimal patient management.

1. Electrocardiogram (ECG):
A non-invasive test that records the electrical activity of the heart is called an electrocardiogram. It provides important information about heart rhythm, conduction abnormalities, and signs of myocardial damage or enlargement. In CHF, an ECG may reveal arrhythmias, conduction disturbances, or evidence of prior myocardial infarction.
It serves as a useful initial screening tool to identify cardiac abnormalities and guide further investigations.

2. Echocardiography:
Echocardiography is a cornerstone diagnostic test in CHF, utilizing sound waves (ultrasound) to create detailed

images of the heart's structure, size, and function. It provides invaluable information about the ventricular dimensions, wall thickness, ejection fraction (EF), valvular abnormalities, and estimates of pulmonary artery pressure. Echocardiography helps assess the overall pumping capacity of the heart, identifies structural abnormalities, and provides insights into the underlying cause of CHF, such as valvular disease or myocardial dysfunction.

3. Chest X-ray:

A chest X-ray is a commonly performed imaging test that provides valuable information about the heart's size, shape, and position. It helps identify signs of fluid accumulation in the lungs, such as pulmonary congestion or pleural effusions.

Additionally, a chest X-ray can reveal an enlarged heart, signs of pulmonary hypertension, or other pulmonary pathologies that may contribute to CHF.

4. Cardiac MRI:

Cardiac magnetic resonance imaging (MRI) provides detailed images of the heart's structure and function using powerful magnets and radio waves. It offers superior visualization of cardiac chambers, myocardial viability, regional wall motion abnormalities, and the presence of scar tissue. Cardiac MRI is particularly useful in assessing ventricular volumes, identifying areas of myocardial scarring or fibrosis, and evaluating complex structural abnormalities that may require surgical intervention.

5. Cardiac CT Scan:

Cardiac computed tomography (CT) scans utilize specialized X-ray techniques to create three-dimensional images of the heart and blood vessels. They can be employed to assess coronary artery disease, identify calcifications or plaques in the coronary arteries, and evaluate the presence of anatomical abnormalities. Cardiac CT scans are especially valuable in determining the need for coronary revascularization procedures and guiding preoperative planning for CHF patients.

6. Blood Tests:

Blood tests play a crucial role in evaluating CHF by measuring specific biomarkers that reflect cardiac stress and damage. Brain natriuretic peptide (BNP) and its N-terminal pro-BNP (NT-proBNP) are commonly measured to assess the severity of heart failure and guide treatment decisions. Other blood tests, such as complete blood count (CBC), renal and liver function tests, and lipid profile, help evaluate associated comorbidities and provide insights into the overall health status of the patient.

7. Exercise Stress Test:

The exercise stress test evaluates the heart's response to physical exertion. It involves monitoring the patient's heart rate, blood pressure, and symptoms during exercise, usually on a treadmill or stationary bike. This test helps assess exercise capacity, identifies exercise-induced symptoms, and evaluates the presence of underlying coronary artery disease or cardiac limitations. Exercise stress testing is particularly useful in determining functional capacity, guiding exercise prescriptions, and assessing response to therapy.

8. Coronary Angiography:

Coronary angiography is an invasive procedure that involves injecting a contrast dye into the coronary arteries to visualize any blockages or narrowing. It is typically performed in patients with suspected coronary artery disease or those who may require revascularization procedures. Coronary angiography provides critical information about the extent and severity of coronary artery disease, allowing for precise treatment planning in CHF patients.

9. Pulmonary Function Tests:

Pulmonary function tests (PFTs) measure lung function and help assess the impact of CHF on pulmonary function. These tests evaluate lung volumes, airflow, and gas exchange and can identify concurrent respiratory conditions or assess the severity of pulmonary involvement in CHF patients.

10. Holter Monitoring and Event Recorders:

Holter monitoring and event recorders are portable devices that continuously record the heart's electrical activity over an extended period. They are particularly useful in detecting and documenting arrhythmias, palpitations, or symptoms that may occur intermittently. These tests provide essential information about heart rhythm disturbances and help guide treatment decisions in CHF patients.

11. Right Heart Catheterization:

Right heart catheterization is an invasive procedure that involves threading a catheter into the right side of the heart to measure pressures and obtain blood samples. It provides direct measurements of central venous pressure, pulmonary artery pressure, cardiac output, and pulmonary capillary wedge pressure.

Right heart catheterization is often reserved for complex cases or when precise hemodynamic data is needed for treatment decisions.

The diagnostic tests and procedures in CHF play a pivotal role in establishing an accurate diagnosis, determining the underlying etiology, assessing disease severity, and guiding therapeutic interventions. By leveraging these comprehensive tools, healthcare professionals can gain invaluable insights into cardiac structure, function, and associated comorbidities, ultimately leading to tailored treatment plans and improved outcomes for CHF patients.

Echocardiogram and Imaging Techniques

Echocardiography and other imaging techniques play a pivotal role in the evaluation of congestive heart failure (CHF), providing valuable insights into cardiac structure, function, and overall cardiovascular health.

In this comprehensive and detailed exploration, we delve into the significance of echocardiography and various imaging techniques in CHF, shedding light on their role in achieving precise assessment and guiding optimal patient management.

1. Echocardiography:

Echocardiography is a non-invasive imaging technique that utilizes high-frequency sound waves (ultrasound) to create detailed images of the heart's structure and function. It is one of the most essential tools in diagnosing and managing CHF. Echocardiography provides a wealth of information, including:

- **Cardiac Chamber Size and Function:** Echocardiography allows for accurate measurement of cardiac chamber dimensions, including the left ventricle (LV) and atria. It provides critical information about LV systolic and diastolic function, assessing parameters such as ejection fraction (EF), fractional shortening, and LV wall motion abnormalities.

- **Valvular Assessment:** Echocardiography enables the evaluation of heart valve structure, function, and any regurgitation or stenosis. It helps identify valvular abnormalities that may contribute to CHF, such as mitral or aortic valve disease.

- **Pulmonary Artery Pressure Estimation:** Echocardiography allows estimation of pulmonary artery pressure by assessing tricuspid regurgitant jet velocity and providing insights into pulmonary hypertension, a common complication in advanced CHF.

- **Tissue Doppler Imaging:** This specialized technique measures myocardial velocities, providing valuable information about regional wall motion abnormalities and assessing the impact of CHF on myocardial function.

- **Strain Imaging:** Strain imaging evaluates myocardial deformation during the cardiac cycle, enabling the detection of subtle changes in myocardial function even before overt dysfunction occurs. It has emerged as a valuable tool in assessing early-stage CHF and monitoring treatment response.

- **Echocardiographic Stress Testing:** Stress echocardiography combines echocardiography with physical or pharmacological stress to evaluate myocardial ischemia, assess contractile reserve, and guide treatment decisions in patients with CHF and suspected coronary artery disease.

2. Cardiac MRI:

Cardiac magnetic resonance imaging (MRI) is a powerful imaging modality that provides highly detailed images of the heart's structure and function. It offers superior spatial resolution and tissue characterization, allowing for a comprehensive assessment of CHF. Cardiac MRI provides valuable information, including:

Ventricular Volumes and Mass: Cardiac MRI accurately measures ventricular volumes, mass, and wall thickness. These measurements help assess ventricular remodeling, chamber dilation, and the impact of CHF on cardiac structure.

- **Tissue Characterization:** Cardiac MRI can differentiate between normal myocardium, scar tissue, and areas of fibrosis or infiltration. This information is crucial for assessing myocardial viability and guiding treatment decisions, such as revascularization procedures or device implantation.

- **Perfusion Imaging:** Cardiac MRI can assess myocardial perfusion by using contrast agents to visualize blood flow within the coronary arteries and detect areas of compromised blood supply. This aids in identifying coronary artery disease and assessing its impact on cardiac function.

- **Late Gadolinium Enhancement:** Late gadolinium enhancement (LGE) imaging is a specialized technique that highlights areas of scar tissue or fibrosis in the myocardium.

It helps identify regions of prior myocardial infarction, non-ischemic cardiomyopathies, or myocarditis, providing critical information for CHF management.

- **4D Flow Imaging:** This advanced technique allows for the visualization and quantification of blood flow patterns in the heart and major vessels. It can identify abnormalities in blood flow dynamics, such as regurgitant or stenotic valves, and assess the impact on cardiac function.

3. Cardiac CT Scan:

Cardiac computed tomography (CT) scan is a non-invasive imaging technique that provides detailed three-dimensional images of the heart and coronary arteries. It offers valuable information in CHF evaluation, including:

- **Coronary Artery Assessment:** Cardiac CT can evaluate the coronary arteries for the presence of plaques, calcifications, or stenosis.

  It helps determine the extent and severity of coronary artery disease and guides treatment decisions, such as revascularization procedures.

- **Cardiac Structure and Function:** Cardiac CT provides detailed images of cardiac chambers, valves, and overall cardiac function. It aids in assessing ventricular volumes, ejection fraction, and detecting structural abnormalities that may contribute to CHF.

- **Pulmonary Venous Assessment:** Cardiac CT can assess the pulmonary veins, providing insights into pulmonary hypertension, pulmonary venous congestion, or abnormalities in pulmonary venous anatomy.

4. Nuclear Imaging:

Nuclear imaging techniques, such as single-photon emission computed tomography (SPECT) or positron emission tomography (PET), can be used to evaluate myocardial perfusion, metabolism, and viability.

These techniques help assess myocardial ischemia, scar tissue, and identify viable myocardium in CHF patients.

These imaging techniques in CHF provide critical information about cardiac structure, function, myocardial viability, and associated complications. They assist in accurate diagnosis, determining the underlying cause of CHF, and guiding treatment decisions. By harnessing the power of echocardiography, cardiac MRI, cardiac CT, and nuclear imaging, healthcare professionals can gain unparalleled insights into the intricacies of CHF, leading to personalized care and improved patient outcomes.

Biomarkers and Laboratory Tests: Decoding Clues for Precise Evaluation

Biomarkers and laboratory tests play a crucial role in the diagnosis, evaluation, and management of congestive heart failure (CHF).

By providing valuable insights into cardiac function, damage, and associated comorbidities, these tests aid in accurate assessment and guide treatment decisions. In this comprehensive exploration, we delve into the significance of biomarkers and laboratory tests in CHF, unraveling their role in decoding vital clues for precise evaluation.

1. Brain Natriuretic Peptide (BNP) and N-terminal pro-BNP (NT-proBNP):

BNP and NT-proBNP are hormones released by the ventricles of the heart in response to increased pressure and stretch, indicating cardiac stress and dysfunction.

These biomarkers serve as valuable indicators of CHF severity and prognosis. Elevated levels of BNP or NT-proBNP in the blood are highly sensitive and specific for the presence of CHF. They help differentiate CHF from other causes of dyspnea and aid in risk stratification, monitoring response to treatment, and guiding therapy adjustments.

2. Cardiac Troponins:

Cardiac troponins are proteins released into the bloodstream when heart muscle cells are damaged or injured, typically as a result of myocardial infarction or myocardial ischemia. While troponin elevation is commonly associated with acute coronary syndromes, it can also occur in CHF due to impaired cardiac function and increased myocardial stress. Elevated troponin levels in CHF patients may indicate underlying myocardial damage or an acute cardiac event and can help guide treatment decisions.

3. Complete Blood Count (CBC):

A complete blood count is a routine laboratory test that provides information about the cellular components of the blood. In CHF, the CBC can reveal anemia, which can contribute to cardiac workload and exacerbate symptoms. Additionally, it helps assess white blood cell count and differential, providing insights into potential infections or inflammatory processes that may affect cardiac function.

4. Renal Function Tests:

Renal function tests, such as serum creatinine and blood urea nitrogen (BUN), assess the kidney's ability to filter waste products from the blood. In CHF, impaired cardiac function can lead to decreased blood flow to the kidneys, resulting in renal dysfunction. Monitoring renal function is essential in managing CHF, as worsening kidney function can further complicate the clinical course and impact treatment decisions.

5. Liver Function Tests:

Liver function tests, including alanine aminotransferase (ALT), aspartate aminotransferase (AST), and bilirubin, provide insights into liver health and function. In CHF, congestion and impaired cardiac output can lead to liver congestion and hepatocellular injury. Elevated liver enzymes and bilirubin levels may indicate hepatic involvement and help assess the severity of CHF.

6. Lipid Profile:

A lipid profile measures cholesterol levels, including total cholesterol, high-density lipoprotein (HDL), low-density lipoprotein (LDL), and triglycerides. While dyslipidemia itself may not be a direct cause of CHF, it is associated with increased cardiovascular risk. Assessing lipid levels helps identify comorbidities and guide treatment strategies, including lifestyle modifications and lipid-lowering medications.

7. Electrolytes and Fluid Balance:

Monitoring electrolyte levels, such as sodium, potassium, and magnesium, is crucial in CHF.

Imbalances in electrolytes can disrupt normal cardiac function and contribute to arrhythmias or exacerbate symptoms. Additionally, evaluating fluid balance through tests like serum osmolality, urine output, and daily weights aids in assessing volume status and guiding diuretic therapy.

8. Thyroid Function Tests:

Thyroid hormones play a crucial role in cardiovascular health and can impact cardiac function. Thyroid dysfunction, including hypothyroidism or hyperthyroidism, can contribute to the development or exacerbation of CHF. Assessing thyroid function through tests such as thyroid-stimulating hormone (TSH), free thyroxine (FT4), and triiodothyronine (T3) levels helps identify underlying thyroid abnormalities that may influence CHF management.

9. Inflammatory and Immunological Markers:

Inflammation and immune system activation play a significant role in the pathophysiology of CHF.

Evaluating markers of inflammation, such as C-reactive protein (CRP) and pro-inflammatory cytokines (e.g., interleukin-6), provides insights into the inflammatory state and helps assess disease severity and prognosis. Additionally, assessing autoimmune markers, such as antinuclear antibodies (ANA), may be warranted in certain cases to explore potential underlying autoimmune conditions contributing to CHF.

10. Genetic Testing:

In specific cases of CHF, genetic testing may be recommended to identify underlying genetic mutations or abnormalities that contribute to the development of cardiac dysfunction. Genetic testing can help determine the etiology of CHF, assess the risk of familial transmission, and guide management strategies, including counseling and targeted therapies.

11. Basic Metabolic Panel (BMP):

The basic metabolic panel includes tests such as blood glucose, electrolytes (sodium, potassium), blood urea nitrogen (BUN), and creatinine.

These tests assess kidney function, fluid and electrolyte balance, and identify any imbalances that may impact CHF management. Abnormalities in electrolyte levels, such as low potassium or high sodium, can affect heart function and fluid balance.

These biomarkers and laboratory tests provide invaluable information about cardiac function, damage, associated comorbidities, and overall disease severity in CHF patients. By leveraging these diagnostic tools, healthcare professionals can gain a comprehensive understanding of the patient's condition, tailor treatment plans, monitor response to therapy, and optimize outcomes in the management of congestive heart failure.

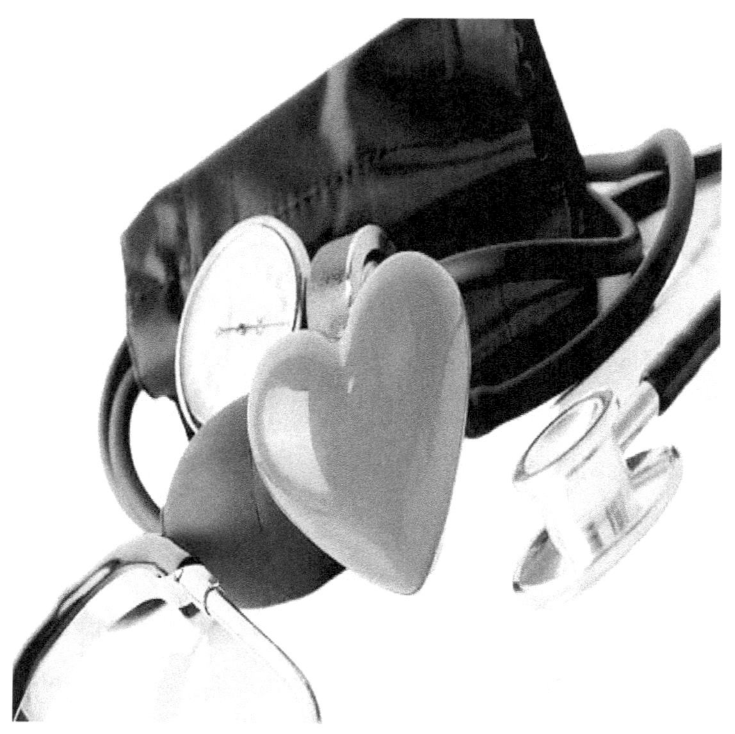

CHAPTER 4

Treatment Approaches: Comprehensive Strategies for Improved Outcomes

Congestive heart failure (CHF) is a complex condition that requires a multifaceted treatment approach to effectively manage symptoms, slow disease progression, and improve overall outcomes. This comprehensive exploration delves into the various treatment approaches for CHF, encompassing lifestyle modifications, medications, surgical interventions, and device therapies. By combining these strategies, healthcare professionals can provide individualized care to optimize the management of congestive heart failure.

1. Lifestyle Modifications:

Lifestyle modifications play a pivotal role in managing CHF and are essential components of treatment. These modifications may include:

- **Sodium Restriction:** Limiting sodium intake helps reduce fluid retention and alleviates symptoms of congestion. Healthcare professionals often recommend a low-sodium diet and provide guidance on reading food labels to identify hidden sources of sodium.

- **Fluid Restriction:** Restricting fluid intake helps maintain fluid balance in CHF patients. Healthcare providers may recommend a daily fluid limit and educate patients on monitoring their fluid intake and recognizing signs of fluid overload.

- **Regular Exercise:** Exercise, tailored to the individual's capabilities, improves cardiovascular fitness, reduces symptoms, and enhances overall well-being.

  Healthcare professionals may prescribe supervised exercise programs or refer patients to cardiac rehabilitation programs.

- **Weight Management:** Achieving and maintaining a healthy weight is crucial in CHF management. Weight monitoring and dietary guidance are essential to prevent fluid retention and exacerbation of symptoms.

- **Smoking Cessation:** Smoking damages the cardiovascular system and worsens CHF symptoms. Encouraging and supporting smoking cessation is vital to reduce the risk of complications and improve overall health.

2. Medications:

Medications are a cornerstone of CHF treatment and aim to improve symptoms, slow disease progression, and reduce hospitalizations. Commonly prescribed medications include:

- **ACE Inhibitors or ARBs:** These medications dilate blood vessels, reduce fluid retention, and improve cardiac function.

- **Beta-Blockers:** Beta-blockers lower heart rate and blood pressure, reducing the workload on the heart and improving overall cardiac function.

- **Diuretics:** Diuretics help eliminate excess fluid and alleviate symptoms of fluid overload, such as edema and shortness of breath.

- **Aldosterone Antagonists:** These medications reduce fluid retention and improve outcomes, particularly in patients with severe CHF.

- **Digoxin:** Digoxin strengthens heart contractions and helps control heart rate in certain cases.

- **Sacubitril/valsartan:** This combination medication enhances beneficial peptides and blocks harmful effects, improving outcomes in CHF with reduced ejection fraction.

3. Surgical Interventions:

In some cases, surgical interventions may be necessary to manage CHF. These may include:

- **Coronary Artery Bypass Grafting (CABG):** CABG surgery is performed to bypass blocked or narrowed coronary arteries, restoring blood flow to the heart muscle.

- **Heart Valve Repair or Replacement:** In CHF patients with valvular heart disease, surgical repair or replacement of damaged heart valves may be necessary to improve cardiac function.

- **Ventricular Assist Devices (VADs):** VADs are mechanical devices implanted in the heart to assist with pumping blood, providing temporary support or serving as a bridge to heart transplantation.

4. Device Therapies:

Device therapies are used to manage specific aspects of CHF and may include:

- **Implantable Cardioverter-Defibrillators (ICDs):** ICDs monitor heart rhythm and deliver electrical shocks if life-threatening arrhythmias occur.

- **Cardiac Resynchronization Therapy (CRT):** CRT involves the implantation of a specialized pacemaker to synchronize the contractions of the heart's chambers, improving overall pumping efficiency.

- **Left Ventricular Assist Devices (LVADs):** LVADs are mechanical pumps that support the heart's pumping function in advanced CHF cases, either as a bridge to transplantation or destination therapy.

5. Palliative and Supportive Care:

In advanced CHF cases where cure or further interventions are not feasible, palliative and supportive care focuses on improving quality of life and providing relief from symptoms. This may involve pain management, emotional support, and assistance with end-of-life planning.

It is important to note that the choice of treatment approach for CHF is individualized based on the patient's specific condition, disease severity, comorbidities, and overall goals of care. Regular monitoring, medication adjustments, and ongoing communication between healthcare providers and patients are vital to optimize treatment outcomes and ensure the best possible quality of life for individuals living with CHF.

In conclusion, the management of congestive heart failure requires a comprehensive treatment approach that encompasses lifestyle modifications, medications, surgical interventions, device therapies, and palliative care. By integrating these strategies, healthcare professionals can provide personalized care, alleviate symptoms, improve cardiac function, and enhance the overall well-being of CHF patients.

Medications for Managing Heart Failure

Effective management of congestive heart failure (CHF) involves a comprehensive approach that includes lifestyle modifications, monitoring fluid balance, and, importantly, the use of medications. Medications play a crucial role in improving symptoms, reducing hospitalizations, and prolonging survival in CHF patients. In this comprehensive exploration, we delve into the various medications used for managing heart failure, shedding light on their mechanisms of action and therapeutic benefits.

1. Angiotensin-Converting Enzyme Inhibitors (ACE inhibitors):

A powerful vasoconstrictor, angiotensin II, is produced when angiotensin I is converted to it by ACE inhibitors. By inhibiting this process, ACE inhibitors dilate blood vessels, reduce fluid retention, and decrease the workload on the heart. These medications improve symptoms, slow disease progression, and reduce mortality rates in CHF patients. Commonly recommended ACE inhibitors include lisinopril, enalapril, and ramipril.

2. Angiotensin Receptor Blockers (ARBs):

ARBs work by blocking the action of angiotensin II on its receptors, thus exerting similar effects as ACE inhibitors. They are typically used as an alternative to ACE inhibitors in patients who cannot tolerate them due to side effects such as persistent cough. ARBs, including losartan, valsartan, and candesartan, are effective in reducing symptoms and improving outcomes in CHF patients.

3. Beta-Blockers:

Beta-blockers inhibit the effects of adrenaline and noradrenaline on the heart, reducing heart rate and blood pressure. These medications improve cardiac function, decrease symptoms, and reduce the risk of hospitalization and mortality in CHF patients. Commonly prescribed beta-blockers for CHF include carvedilol, metoprolol succinate, and bisoprolol.

4. Diuretics:

Diuretics, such as furosemide and hydrochlorothiazide, are used to reduce fluid retention and alleviate symptoms of congestion in CHF patients.

They promote diuresis by increasing urine production and decreasing fluid volume overload. Diuretics provide relief from symptoms like edema and shortness of breath and help maintain fluid balance.

5. Aldosterone Antagonists:

Aldosterone antagonists, such as spironolactone and eplerenone, inhibit the effects of aldosterone, a hormone that promotes fluid and sodium retention.

These medications reduce fluid overload, improve symptoms, and decrease the risk of hospitalization and mortality in CHF patients, particularly in those with more severe disease.

6. Digoxin:

Digoxin is a medication derived from the foxglove plant and has been used for many years in the management of CHF. It strengthens the force of heart contractions, slows the heart rate, and improves symptoms in patients with systolic heart failure. Digoxin is typically reserved for patients with persistent symptoms despite optimal therapy or those with atrial fibrillation.

7. Ivabradine:

Ivabradine is a newer medication that specifically targets the heart's sinus node, reducing heart rate without affecting blood pressure. It is indicated for patients with symptomatic heart failure and reduced ejection fraction who are already receiving guideline-directed medical therapy. Ivabradine helps improve symptoms, reduce hospitalizations, and enhance exercise tolerance.

8. Sacubitril/Valsartan:

Sacubitril/valsartan is a combination medication that combines a neprilysin inhibitor (sacubitril) with an angiotensin receptor blocker (valsartan). It enhances the body's natural protective mechanisms by increasing levels of beneficial peptides and blocking the harmful effects of angiotensin II. Sacubitril/valsartan is indicated for patients with heart failure with reduced ejection fraction and has shown significant benefits in reducing hospitalizations and mortality.

9. Antiplatelet and Anticoagulant Medications:

In CHF patients with comorbid conditions like atrial fibrillation or coronary artery disease, antiplatelet and anticoagulant medications may be prescribed to prevent blood clots and reduce the risk of stroke or myocardial infarction.

It is important to note that the specific choice of medications and their dosages may vary based on individual patient characteristics, disease severity, and comorbidities.

The management of CHF requires close collaboration between healthcare providers and patients to optimize medication regimens and ensure regular monitoring for efficacy and potential side effects.

In conclusion, medications play a crucial role in the management of congestive heart failure. They help alleviate symptoms, improve cardiac function, and reduce the risk of complications and mortality.

By tailoring medication regimens to individual patients and closely monitoring their response, healthcare professionals can optimize treatment outcomes and enhance the quality of life for individuals living with CHF.

Lifestyle Modifications and Self-Care

In addition to medical interventions, lifestyle modifications and self-care practices play a vital role in the management of congestive heart failure (CHF).

These proactive measures empower patients to take control of their health, reduce symptoms, enhance overall well-being, and improve outcomes. Here, we explore comprehensive lifestyle modifications and self-care strategies that can support individuals with CHF in their journey toward a healthier and more fulfilling life.

1. Diet and Nutrition:

- **Sodium Restriction:** Limiting sodium intake is crucial in managing CHF.

Patients are advised to reduce their consumption of processed and packaged foods, which often contain high amounts of sodium. Instead, emphasizing fresh fruits, vegetables, whole grains, lean proteins, and low-sodium alternatives can help maintain fluid balance and alleviate symptoms of fluid retention.

- **Fluid Management:** Monitoring fluid intake is essential in CHF. Patients should work with healthcare professionals to determine a suitable daily fluid allowance based on their individual needs. This includes considering both beverages and foods with high water content.

- **Heart-Healthy Eating:** Adopting a heart-healthy diet rich in fruits, vegetables, whole grains, lean proteins, and low-fat dairy products can support overall cardiovascular health.

Patients are encouraged to consult with registered dietitians or nutritionists to develop personalized meal plans that align with their specific dietary requirements and restrictions.

2. Physical Activity and Exercise:

- **Regular Exercise:** Engaging in regular physical activity is beneficial for CHF patients. Moderate aerobic exercise, as recommended by healthcare providers, can improve cardiovascular fitness, reduce symptoms, enhance circulation, and increase energy levels. Patients should consult their healthcare team for guidance on appropriate exercise programs and intensity levels.

- **Cardiac Rehabilitation:** Cardiac rehabilitation programs provide structured exercise training, education, and support for individuals with cardiovascular conditions, including CHF.

These programs are supervised by healthcare professionals and can help patients safely and effectively increase their exercise capacity while providing important education on heart-healthy habits.

3. Smoking Cessation:

- Quitting smoking is crucial for individuals with CHF. Smoking damages blood vessels, increases blood pressure, and impairs lung function, exacerbating symptoms and worsening the progression of the disease. Healthcare professionals can provide resources, support, and smoking cessation strategies to help patients successfully quit smoking.

4. Medication Adherence:

- Strict adherence to prescribed medications is essential for CHF management.

Patients should follow medication schedules, adhere to recommended dosages, and communicate any concerns or side effects to their healthcare providers. Medications prescribed for CHF, such as ACE inhibitors, beta-blockers, and diuretics, are integral to symptom relief and slowing disease progression.

5. Stress Management and Emotional Well-being:

- Stress reduction techniques, such as meditation, deep breathing exercises, and mindfulness practices, can help manage stress and promote emotional well-being. Engaging in activities that bring joy and relaxation, such as hobbies, socializing, and spending time in nature, can also contribute to improved overall mental health.

6. Regular Monitoring:

- Regular monitoring of weight, blood pressure, and symptoms is crucial for individuals with CHF.

Patients should keep track of their weight, aiming to report any significant fluctuations to their healthcare team. Monitoring blood pressure at home, as advised by healthcare providers, can help manage hypertension, a common comorbidity of CHF. Additionally, staying vigilant about changes in symptoms, such as increased shortness of breath or swelling, can help identify exacerbations and allow for timely intervention.

7. Education and Support:

- Education plays a pivotal role in empowering individuals with CHF to manage their condition effectively. Healthcare professionals should provide comprehensive education on CHF, its symptoms, medications, and lifestyle modifications. Support groups and community resources can also provide valuable emotional support and practical tips for self-care.

In conclusion, lifestyle modifications and self-care practices are integral components of managing congestive heart failure. By adopting a heart-healthy diet, engaging in regular exercise, quitting smoking, adhering to prescribed medications, managing stress, and monitoring their condition, patients can actively participate in their own care and experience improved quality of life. Collaboration between healthcare professionals and patients is crucial to developing personalized self-care plans and empowering individuals with CHF to take control of their health journey.

Dietary Changes and Fluid Restriction

Dietary modifications are crucial in the management of congestive heart failure (CHF). By adopting a heart-healthy eating plan and implementing fluid restriction strategies, individuals with CHF can help alleviate symptoms, manage fluid balance, and support overall cardiovascular health.

Here, we delve into comprehensive dietary changes and fluid restriction practices that can optimize the management of CHF.

1. Sodium Restriction:

Reducing sodium intake is of paramount importance for individuals with CHF. Excess sodium can lead to fluid retention, worsen congestion, and strain the heart. Here are key strategies for sodium restriction:

- **Limit Processed and Packaged Foods:** Many processed and packaged foods are very high in sodium. It's important to read food labels and select low-sodium alternatives whenever possible. Opt for fresh, whole foods and prepare meals at home to have greater control over sodium content.

- **Avoid Added Salt:** Minimize the use of table salt and avoid adding salt to dishes during cooking or at the table. Instead, enhance flavors with herbs, spices, and low-sodium seasoning blends.

- **Choose Low-Sodium Options:** Opt for low-sodium or sodium-free versions of condiments, sauces, and canned goods. Look for products labeled as "low-sodium," "no salt added," or "unsalted."

- **Be Mindful of Hidden Sodium:** Be aware of hidden sources of sodium, such as deli meats, canned soups, fast food, and restaurant meals. Ask for nutrition information or look for lower-sodium options when dining out.

- **Fresh Fruits and Vegetables:** Emphasize a diet rich in fresh fruits and vegetables, as they are naturally low in sodium and provide essential nutrients and fiber.

2. Fluid Restriction:

Fluid management is crucial for individuals with CHF to prevent fluid overload and maintain optimal fluid balance.

Here are strategies for fluid restriction:

- Collaborate with Healthcare Team: Work closely with your healthcare team to determine an appropriate daily fluid allowance based on your individual needs and medical condition. This may include considering both beverages and foods with high water content.

- **Monitor Fluid Intake:** Keep track of your fluid intake throughout the day. Measure and record the amount of fluids consumed, including water, beverages, soups, and foods with high water content like fruits and vegetables.

- **Set Fluid Goals:** Establish specific fluid goals recommended by your healthcare team and aim to adhere to them consistently. This may involve dividing your daily fluid allowance into smaller portions to be consumed at specific intervals.

- **Choose Fluid Alternatives:** Opt for low-sodium or sodium-free beverages. Avoid or limit high-sodium beverages such as sodas, sports drinks, and commercially packaged fruit juices. Unsweetened herbal teas, flavored water, and small amounts of low-fat milk can be hydrating options.

- **Be Mindful of Liquid Consistency:** Pay attention to the consistency of foods that are high in water content, such as soups, stews, and ice cream. These contribute to overall fluid intake and should be factored into your daily allowance.

- **Manage Thirst Sensations:** If you experience feelings of thirst, try rinsing your mouth with cold water, sucking on ice chips, or consuming small amounts of moist foods to help alleviate the sensation without exceeding your fluid limits.

- **Consult with Healthcare Professionals:** Regularly communicate with your healthcare team to review and adjust fluid restrictions as needed based on changes in your condition or medication regimen.

Remember, it is crucial to individualize dietary changes and fluid restrictions based on your specific needs, health status, and recommendations from your healthcare team. Adhering to these modifications, along with other aspects of CHF management, can help optimize fluid balance, alleviate symptoms, and promote overall cardiovascular health.

Exercise and Rehabilitation Programs

Exercise and rehabilitation programs are essential components of the management of congestive heart failure (CHF).

Engaging in regular physical activity under the guidance of healthcare professionals can improve cardiovascular fitness, enhance functional capacity, reduce symptoms, and improve overall well-being for individuals living with CHF.

Here, we explore comprehensive exercise and rehabilitation strategies that can empower patients and promote optimal heart health.

1. Importance of Exercise in CHF Management:

Regular exercise offers numerous benefits for individuals with CHF. It improves cardiac function, increases exercise tolerance, strengthens the heart muscle, enhances circulation, and helps manage comorbidities such as hypertension and obesity. Moreover, exercise can positively impact mental health, reduce stress, and improve quality of life. However, it is crucial to consult with healthcare professionals before initiating any exercise program to ensure safety and appropriateness for individual needs.

2. Cardiac Rehabilitation Programs:

Cardiac rehabilitation programs provide structured exercise training, education, and support for individuals with cardiovascular conditions, including CHF. These programs are typically conducted in a supervised setting, such as a hospital or specialized clinic, under the guidance of a multidisciplinary team of healthcare professionals. Key components of cardiac rehabilitation programs include:

- **Exercise Training:** Cardiac rehabilitation programs involve individualized exercise prescriptions tailored to each patient's specific needs and abilities. The exercise regimen typically includes aerobic activities, such as walking, cycling, or swimming, as well as resistance training to improve muscle strength. Exercise sessions are monitored to ensure safety and optimize training intensity.

- **Education and Risk Factor Modification:** Cardiac rehabilitation programs provide education on heart-healthy lifestyle modifications, including dietary changes, medication adherence, stress management, and smoking cessation. Patients receive guidance on managing risk factors, understanding their medications, and recognizing warning signs or symptoms that require medical attention.

- **Psychological Support:** Emotional well-being plays a vital role in CHF management. Cardiac rehabilitation programs often include psychological support, such as counseling or stress management techniques, to address the psychological impact of CHF and promote mental well-being.

- **Lifestyle and Behavior Modification:** Cardiac rehabilitation programs help patients make sustainable lifestyle changes by providing resources, guidance, and strategies to support behavior modification.

  This may involve setting realistic goals, developing action plans, and fostering self-management skills to promote long-term adherence to heart-healthy habits.

3. Supervised Exercise Training:

For individuals with CHF who do not have access to cardiac rehabilitation programs, supervised exercise training can still be beneficial. Working with healthcare professionals, such as exercise physiologists or cardiac rehabilitation specialists, allows for personalized exercise prescriptions and ongoing monitoring to ensure safety and optimize exercise intensity.

4. Home Exercise Programs:

In cases where supervised exercise programs are not feasible, healthcare professionals can develop home exercise programs tailored to individual needs and capabilities. These programs typically involve aerobic activities, such as walking or stationary cycling, along with resistance exercises using body weight or resistance bands. Patients are provided with guidance on exercise duration, frequency, and intensity to ensure a safe and effective workout.

5. Precautions and Monitoring:

When engaging in exercise, individuals with CHF should be aware of certain precautions and monitoring practices:

- **Regular Medical Evaluation:** It is essential to undergo regular medical evaluations to assess the safety and suitability of exercise programs. Healthcare professionals can monitor changes in cardiac function, adjust medications if necessary, and provide guidance on exercise modifications.

- **Monitoring Exercise Intensity:** Monitoring exercise intensity using methods like heart rate monitoring or the Rating of Perceived Exertion (RPE) scale can help individuals with CHF ensure they are exercising within a safe and appropriate range.

- **Listening to the Body:** It is crucial to pay attention to the body's signals during exercise. Individuals with CHF should be aware of any symptoms or warning signs, such as chest pain, excessive shortness of breath, dizziness, or abnormal heart rhythms, and consult with their healthcare team if these symptoms occur.

- **Gradual Progression:** Exercise programs should be gradually progressed over time to avoid excessive strain on the cardiovascular system. Gradual increases in exercise duration, intensity, or resistance allow the body to adapt and strengthen without overexertion.

In conclusion, exercise and rehabilitation programs play a significant role in the management of congestive heart failure. These programs improve cardiovascular fitness, enhance functional capacity, and promote overall well-being for individuals living with CHF.

Whether through cardiac rehabilitation programs, supervised exercise training, or home exercise programs, healthcare professionals can provide guidance, support, and monitoring to ensure safe and effective participation in exercise. By incorporating exercise as part of a comprehensive treatment plan, individuals with CHF can strengthen their hearts and improve their quality of life.

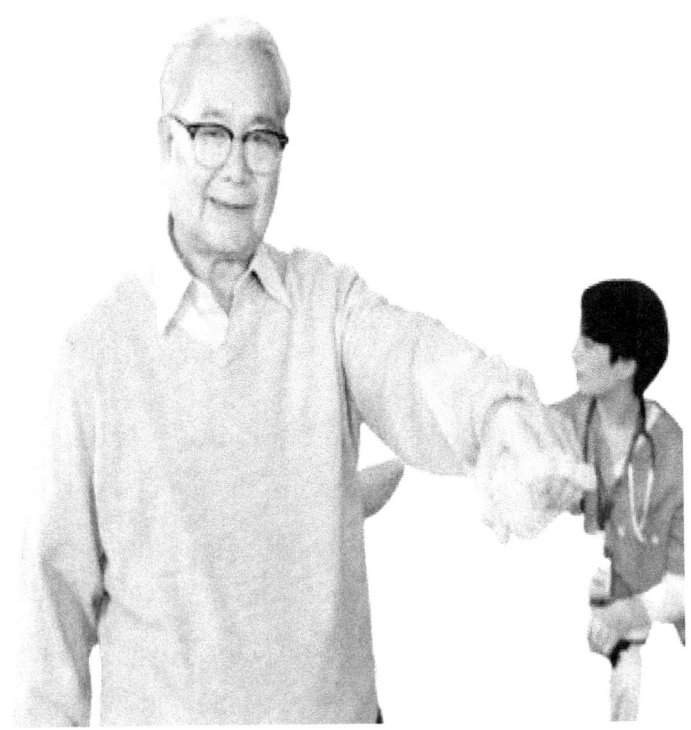

CHAPTER 5

Advanced Congestive Heart Failure Therapies and Treatments

While lifestyle modifications, medications, and conventional treatments form the cornerstone of congestive heart failure (CHF) management, advanced treatments and therapies have emerged to provide additional options for individuals with more severe or advanced stages of the condition. These cutting-edge interventions aim to enhance heart function, alleviate symptoms, and improve overall quality of life. In this comprehensive guide, we explore the most notable advanced treatments and therapies for CHF.

1. Implantable Cardioverter-Defibrillator (ICD):

ICDs are electronic devices implanted under the skin to continuously monitor heart rhythms.

These devices can deliver an electric shock if a life-threatening arrhythmia is detected, restoring normal heart rhythm and preventing sudden cardiac arrest. ICDs are typically recommended for individuals with a history of life-threatening arrhythmias or those at high risk of sudden cardiac death.

2. Cardiac Resynchronization Therapy (CRT):

CRT, also known as biventricular pacing, involves the placement of a specialized pacemaker that coordinates the timing of electrical impulses to improve the synchronization of the heart's chambers. By stimulating the heart's ventricles simultaneously, CRT can enhance pumping efficiency, optimize cardiac output, and alleviate symptoms such as shortness of breath and fatigue. CRT is typically recommended for individuals with certain types of heart failure, particularly those with a reduced ejection fraction and evidence of ventricular dyssynchrony.

3. Ventricular Assist Devices (VAD):

VADs are mechanical devices implanted in individuals with severe heart failure to assist or replace the pumping function of the heart. These devices can be used as a bridge to transplantation or as long-term therapy for individuals who are not eligible for a heart transplant. VADs can significantly improve quality of life, increase exercise tolerance, and prolong survival for individuals with advanced heart failure.

4. Heart Transplantation:

The only effective treatment for end-stage heart failure is heart transplantation. It involves the surgical replacement of a diseased heart with a healthy heart from a donor. Heart transplantation can offer a new lease on life for individuals with severe CHF who have exhausted other treatment options. However, due to the limited availability of donor hearts, strict eligibility criteria, and the need for lifelong immunosuppressive medications, heart transplantation is reserved for select patients.

5. MitraClip Procedure:

The MitraClip procedure is a minimally invasive catheter-based intervention used to treat mitral valve regurgitation, a common complication of heart failure. It involves the placement of a small device that clips the edges of the mitral valve together, reducing the backflow of blood and improving overall valve function. The MitraClip procedure is typically considered for individuals with significant mitral valve regurgitation who are not suitable candidates for surgical valve repair or replacement.

6. Left Ventricular Assist Devices (LVAD):

LVADs are mechanical devices that provide long-term support to the left ventricle, the main pumping chamber of the heart. These devices can be used as a bridge to transplantation or as destination therapy for individuals who are not eligible for heart transplantation. LVADs improve blood flow, relieve symptoms, and extend survival for individuals with advanced heart failure.

7. Regenerative Therapies:

Regenerative therapies hold promise in the field of heart failure management. These therapies aim to repair or regenerate damaged heart tissue, restore cardiac function, and potentially reduce the need for transplantation. Stem cell therapy, gene therapy, and tissue engineering are among the innovative approaches being explored in clinical trials and research studies.

8. Pharmacological Innovations:

Continual advancements in pharmacotherapy have resulted in new medications that target specific pathways involved in heart failure progression. These include angiotensin receptor-neprilysin inhibitors (ARNIs), sodium-glucose cotransporter-2 inhibitors (SGLT2 inhibitors), and other novel agents that have demonstrated efficacy in reducing hospitalizations, improving symptoms, and prolonging survival in individuals with heart failure.

It is important to note that the eligibility and appropriateness of advanced treatments and therapies for CHF vary based on individual patient factors, disease severity, and the recommendations of a multidisciplinary heart failure team. Consultation with cardiovascular specialists, including heart failure specialists and cardiac surgeons, is essential to determine the most appropriate treatment approach for each individual.

In conclusion, advanced treatments and therapies offer new avenues of hope for individuals with congestive heart failure. From implantable devices and surgical interventions to regenerative therapies and pharmacological innovations, these cutting-edge approaches aim to enhance heart function, alleviate symptoms, and improve quality of life for individuals living with advanced stages of CHF. As research continues to advance, the future holds even greater promise for transforming the landscape of congestive heart failure management.

Implantable Devices (Pacemakers and Defibrillators) for Congestive Heart Failure

Implantable devices, such as pacemakers and defibrillators, have revolutionized the management of congestive heart failure (CHF). These advanced technologies are designed to regulate heart rhythms, improve cardiac function, and prevent life-threatening arrhythmias. In this comprehensive guide, we delve into the details of pacemakers and defibrillators as key implantable devices used in CHF treatment.

1. Pacemakers:

Pacemakers are small electronic devices implanted beneath the skin, usually in the chest area, to regulate and maintain the heart's rhythm.

They consist of two main components: a generator (containing a battery and circuitry) and leads (thin, insulated wires) that connect the generator to the heart. Pacemakers are primarily used to treat bradycardia, a condition characterized by a slow heart rate or irregular heart rhythms that can lead to symptoms such as fatigue, dizziness, and fainting.

Key features and functions of pacemakers include:

- **Sensing:** Pacemakers continuously monitor the heart's electrical signals to detect abnormalities or pauses in the heart rhythm. They sense the heart's own electrical activity and determine when to deliver electrical impulses.

- **Pacing:** When the pacemaker detects a slow or irregular heart rhythm, it delivers small electrical impulses to stimulate the heart muscle, initiating a heartbeat and maintaining an optimal heart rate.

- **Rate-Responsive Pacing:** Some pacemakers have the ability to adjust the heart rate based on the body's needs.

They can increase the heart rate during physical activity and decrease it during rest, allowing for a more natural response to exertion.

- **Dual-Chamber and Biventricular Pacing:** Advanced pacemakers can synchronize the contractions of the heart's chambers (atria and ventricles) to optimize pumping efficiency. Dual-chamber pacemakers coordinate the timing of electrical impulses between the atria and ventricles, while biventricular pacemakers, also known as cardiac resynchronization therapy (CRT) pacemakers, coordinate the electrical impulses between the right and left ventricles, improving overall heart function.

2. Implantable Cardioverter-Defibrillators (ICDs):

ICDs are implantable devices that not only regulate heart rhythms but also have the capability to deliver life-saving shocks when a life-threatening arrhythmia, such as ventricular fibrillation or ventricular tachycardia, is detected.

ICDs are typically recommended for individuals at high risk of sudden cardiac death due to a history of arrhythmias or certain structural heart conditions.

Key features and functions of ICDs include:

- **Sensing and Monitoring:** Like pacemakers, ICDs continuously monitor the heart's electrical signals for abnormal rhythms. They can differentiate between benign and potentially life-threatening arrhythmias.

- **Defibrillation:** When an ICD detects a life-threatening arrhythmia, it delivers a high-energy electrical shock (defibrillation) to restore normal heart rhythm. This shock interrupts the abnormal electrical activity and allows the heart to resume a regular rhythm.

- **Antitachycardia Pacing (ATP):** In addition to defibrillation, ICDs can also deliver rapid pacing impulses, known as ATP, to terminate certain fast arrhythmias without the need for a high-energy shock.

- **Monitoring and Data Storage:** ICDs can store valuable data on the heart's electrical activity and arrhythmia occurrences. This information can be accessed by healthcare professionals during follow-up appointments to assess device function, evaluate arrhythmia management, and make any necessary adjustments to the device programming.

Both pacemakers and ICDs are implanted through a minor surgical procedure performed by a cardiologist or cardiac electrophysiologist. The procedure involves making a small incision, typically in the upper chest, and guiding the leads to the heart through a vein. The generator is then implanted under the skin, usually in the upper chest or abdomen, and connected to the leads.

The entire process is performed under local anesthesia, and patients are often able to resume their normal activities within a few days.

It is important to note that the decision to implant a pacemaker or ICD is based on individual patient characteristics, specific heart rhythm abnormalities, and the recommendations of a multidisciplinary heart failure team. Regular follow-up appointments are necessary to monitor device function, optimize programming settings, and ensure the ongoing effectiveness of the implanted device.

In conclusion, pacemakers and ICDs have transformed the management of congestive heart failure by regulating heart rhythms, improving cardiac function, and preventing life-threatening arrhythmias. These implantable devices provide a vital lifeline for individuals with CHF, enhancing their quality of life and reducing the risk of sudden cardiac death. With ongoing advancements in technology, these devices continue to evolve, offering improved features and more personalized therapy options for individuals living with CHF.

Cardiac Resynchronization Therapy (CRT) for Congestive Heart Failure Treatment

Congestive heart failure (CHF) is a complex condition that often involves impaired coordination and synchronization of the heart's pumping chambers, leading to reduced cardiac output and debilitating symptoms. Cardiac Resynchronization Therapy (CRT) is an advanced treatment approach designed to improve the coordination and function of the heart in individuals with certain types of heart failure. In this comprehensive guide, we explore the intricacies of CRT, its benefits, and its role in the management of congestive heart failure.

1. Understanding Cardiac Resynchronization Therapy (CRT):

CRT, also known as biventricular pacing, involves the use of specialized pacemakers to improve the synchronization of the heart's chambers.

It aims to coordinate the timing of electrical impulses to enhance pumping efficiency, optimize cardiac output, and alleviate symptoms associated with heart failure. CRT is primarily recommended for individuals with specific types of heart failure, particularly those with a reduced ejection fraction and evidence of ventricular dyssynchrony.

2. How CRT Works:

CRT devices consist of a small generator (pacemaker) and leads (thin wires) that are implanted in the heart. The leads are positioned in the right atrium, right ventricle, and left ventricle to deliver electrical impulses to the heart's chambers. The pacing impulses from the CRT device synchronize the contractions of the ventricles, improving the coordination and efficiency of the heart's pumping action.

3. Benefits of CRT:

a. Enhanced Pumping Efficiency: By synchronizing the contractions of the ventricles, CRT improves the coordination of the heart's pumping action, leading to increased cardiac output and better circulation of oxygenated blood throughout the body.

b. Symptom Relief: CRT can alleviate symptoms associated with congestive heart failure, such as shortness of breath, fatigue, and exercise intolerance. Improved heart function and circulation result in enhanced exercise capacity and overall quality of life.

c. Reverse Remodeling: CRT has been shown to promote reverse remodeling, which refers to the improvement in the structure and function of the heart. It can lead to a reduction in ventricular size, improved cardiac muscle function, and potentially halt or reverse the progression of heart failure.

d. Reduced Hospitalizations and Mortality: Numerous studies have demonstrated that CRT reduces the risk of heart failure-related hospitalizations and mortality rates in eligible patients.

4. Eligibility for CRT:

CRT is typically considered for individuals who meet specific criteria, including:

- Moderate to severe heart failure symptoms (NYHA class II-IV) despite optimal medical therapy
- Reduced ejection fraction (typically $\leq 35\%$)
- Evidence of ventricular dyssynchrony, assessed through echocardiography or other imaging techniques

5. Implantation Procedure:

CRT implantation is performed by a skilled cardiac electrophysiologist. The procedure involves making a small incision, usually in the upper chest area, and placing the leads in the heart's chambers. The generator is then implanted under the skin, typically in the upper chest or abdomen.

The procedure is performed under local anesthesia, and patients are often able to resume their normal activities within a few days.

6. Follow-up and Device Optimization:

Following CRT implantation, regular follow-up appointments are essential to monitor device function, optimize programming settings, and evaluate the patient's response to therapy.

Adjustments to pacing parameters may be made to ensure optimal synchronization and maximize the benefits of CRT.

7. Additional Advances in CRT:

Recent advancements in CRT technology have led to the development of multisite pacing and quadripolar leads, allowing for more precise positioning of the pacing electrodes and improved response to therapy. These advances aim to further enhance the effectiveness of CRT in eligible patients.

In conclusion, Cardiac Resynchronization Therapy (CRT) offers a significant advancement in the treatment of congestive heart failure. By synchronizing the contractions of the heart's chambers, CRT improves pumping efficiency, reduces symptoms, and enhances the quality of life for individuals living with heart failure. As technology continues to evolve and more personalized approaches emerge, CRT remains a valuable tool in the comprehensive management of congestive heart failure, offering renewed hope and improved outcomes for eligible patients.

Ventricular Assist Devices (VADs) for Congestive Heart Failure Treatment

Congestive heart failure (CHF) is a complex condition that can progress to an advanced stage where conventional medical therapies may no longer be sufficient. In such cases, Ventricular Assist Devices (VADs) offer a lifeline by providing mechanical support to the failing heart.

In this comprehensive guide, we explore the intricacies of VADs, their benefits, and their role in the management of congestive heart failure.

1. Understanding Ventricular Assist Devices (VADs):

VADs are implantable mechanical pumps designed to assist or replace the function of a weakened or failing ventricle in the heart. These devices are typically used in two main ways: as a bridge to heart transplantation or as long-term support for individuals who are not eligible for transplantation. VADs can be implanted in one or both ventricles, depending on the specific needs of the patient.

2. Types of VADs:

a. Left Ventricular Assist Devices (LVADs): LVADs are the most common type of VAD and are used to support the left ventricle, which is responsible for pumping oxygenated blood to the body. These devices are implanted to augment or replace the pumping function of the left ventricle, thereby improving cardiac output and alleviating symptoms associated with heart failure.

b. Right Ventricular Assist Devices (RVADs): RVADs are less common and are used to support the right ventricle, which pumps deoxygenated blood to the lungs for oxygenation. RVADs are typically used in conjunction with LVADs in cases where both ventricles require mechanical support.

c. Biventricular Assist Devices (BiVADs): BiVADs provide support to both the left and right ventricles simultaneously. They are typically used in severe cases of biventricular heart failure, where both ventricles are significantly weakened.

3. Benefits of VADs:

a. Improved Cardiac Output: VADs significantly improve cardiac output by assisting or taking over the pumping function of the failing ventricle(s). This results in better circulation of oxygenated blood throughout the body, alleviating symptoms such as fatigue, shortness of breath, and fluid retention.

b. Bridge to Transplantation: VADs can serve as a bridge to heart transplantation, providing mechanical support while a suitable donor heart becomes available. This helps to stabilize the patient's condition, improve their overall health, and increase the chances of a successful transplant.

c. Destination Therapy: In cases where heart transplantation is not feasible or desired, VADs can serve as long-term therapy, providing ongoing support and improving the quality of life for individuals with end-stage heart failure.

d. Potential for Recovery: In some cases, VADs may allow the native heart to rest and recover its function over time.

This can lead to a significant improvement in heart function and, in some instances, the possibility of device removal.

4. Implantation Procedure:

VAD implantation is a complex surgical procedure performed by a multidisciplinary team of cardiac surgeons and cardiologists.

The surgery involves making an incision in the chest to access the heart, attaching the VAD's inflow and outflow cannulas to the appropriate ventricles, and connecting them to the external power source and control unit. The patient is typically placed on a heart-lung machine during the procedure to maintain circulation and oxygenation.

5. Post-Implantation Care and Management:

Following VAD implantation, patients require close monitoring and specialized care. This includes regular follow-up visits, device checks, and adjustments to optimize device settings. Patients and their caregivers receive thorough training on device operation, maintenance, and potential complications.

6. Potential Complications and Risks:

While VADs can significantly improve the quality of life for individuals with congestive heart failure, they also carry certain risks and complications.

These may include infections, bleeding, device malfunction, blood clot formation, and adverse reactions to anticoagulant medications. Regular monitoring and prompt intervention can help reduce these risks.

7. Ongoing Advances in VAD Technology:

The field of VADs continues to evolve rapidly, with ongoing advancements in device technology, miniaturization, and long-term reliability. Efforts are being made to develop fully implantable VADs, improve battery life, and enhance patient mobility and quality of life.

In conclusion, Ventricular Assist Devices (VADs) have revolutionized the management of advanced congestive heart failure. Whether as a bridge to transplantation or as long-term support, VADs offer a life-saving therapy option for individuals with failing hearts.

As technology advances and experience grows, VADs continue to provide hope, improve outcomes, and offer a second chance at life for those living with advanced congestive heart failure.

Heart Transplantation for Congestive Heart Failure

Congestive heart failure (CHF) in its advanced stages can severely impact the quality of life and prognosis of individuals. For those who have exhausted all other treatment options, heart transplantation offers a potential cure and a chance at a new lease on life. In this comprehensive guide, we delve into the intricacies of heart transplantation, its benefits, and its role in the management of congestive heart failure.

1. Understanding Heart Transplantation:

Heart transplantation involves replacing a diseased or failing heart with a healthy donor heart from a deceased individual.

It is considered the gold standard treatment for end-stage congestive heart failure when other therapies, such as medication, lifestyle modifications, and device therapies, have been maximized but no longer provide adequate support.

2. The Transplant Process:

a. Evaluation and Waitlist: Individuals undergoing heart transplantation undergo a comprehensive evaluation process to determine their suitability for transplantation. This includes a thorough assessment of their medical history, physical condition, and other factors such as age, overall health, and compatibility. If deemed eligible, patients are placed on a waiting list for a suitable donor heart.

b. Donor Selection and Organ Allocation: The process of matching a suitable donor heart to a recipient involves various factors, including blood type, body size, urgency, and time spent on the waiting list. Organ procurement organizations (OPOs) facilitate the allocation process and ensure fair distribution based on established criteria.

c. Surgery and Transplantation: Once a suitable donor heart becomes available, the transplantation surgery takes place. The recipient's diseased heart is carefully removed, and the donor heart is implanted, connecting it to the recipient's blood vessels and ensuring proper function.

The surgery is performed by a skilled cardiac surgical team under general anesthesia.

3. Benefits of Heart Transplantation:

a. Improved Quality of Life: Heart transplantation can significantly improve the quality of life for individuals with end-stage congestive heart failure. Symptoms such as fatigue, shortness of breath, and exercise intolerance often diminish, allowing recipients to engage in activities they were previously unable to enjoy.

b. Prolonged Life Expectancy: Heart transplantation offers a significant increase in life expectancy for eligible candidates. While individual outcomes may vary, the average survival rate after heart transplantation is generally favorable, with many recipients living 10 years or longer.

c. Restoration of Cardiac Function: Heart transplantation provides a functioning, healthy heart that can effectively pump blood throughout the body, restoring normal cardiac function and alleviating the symptoms of congestive heart failure.

4. Post-Transplant Care:

After heart transplantation, recipients require lifelong follow-up care to ensure the success of the procedure and minimize the risk of complications. This includes close monitoring of the transplanted heart's function, regular check-ups, immunosuppressive medications to prevent organ rejection, and adopting a healthy lifestyle to maintain overall well-being.

5. Potential Challenges and Considerations:

a. Organ Shortage: The demand for donor hearts far exceeds the available supply, leading to a significant shortage of organs. This underscores the importance of increasing awareness about organ donation and exploring alternative strategies such as mechanical circulatory support devices as a bridge to transplantation.

b. Immunosuppression: To prevent rejection of the transplanted heart, recipients must take immunosuppressive medications. These medications weaken the immune system, which can increase the risk of infections and other complications. Close monitoring and adherence to medication regimens are crucial for long-term success.

c. Lifestyle Changes: Following heart transplantation, recipients are encouraged to adopt a healthy lifestyle, including regular exercise, a balanced diet, and avoiding factors that may negatively impact the transplanted heart's health, such as smoking and excessive intake of alcohol.

6. Ongoing Advances in Heart Transplantation:

Heart transplantation is a constantly evolving field, with ongoing research and technological advancements aimed at improving outcomes and expanding the donor pool. This includes innovations in organ preservation, immunosuppressive therapies, and the development of strategies to address organ shortage challenges.

In conclusion, heart transplantation is a life-saving treatment option for individuals with end-stage congestive heart failure. It offers the potential for an improved quality of life, increased life expectancy, and restoration of cardiac function.

With ongoing advancements and increased awareness about organ donation, heart transplantation continues to provide hope and a second chance at life for those in need.

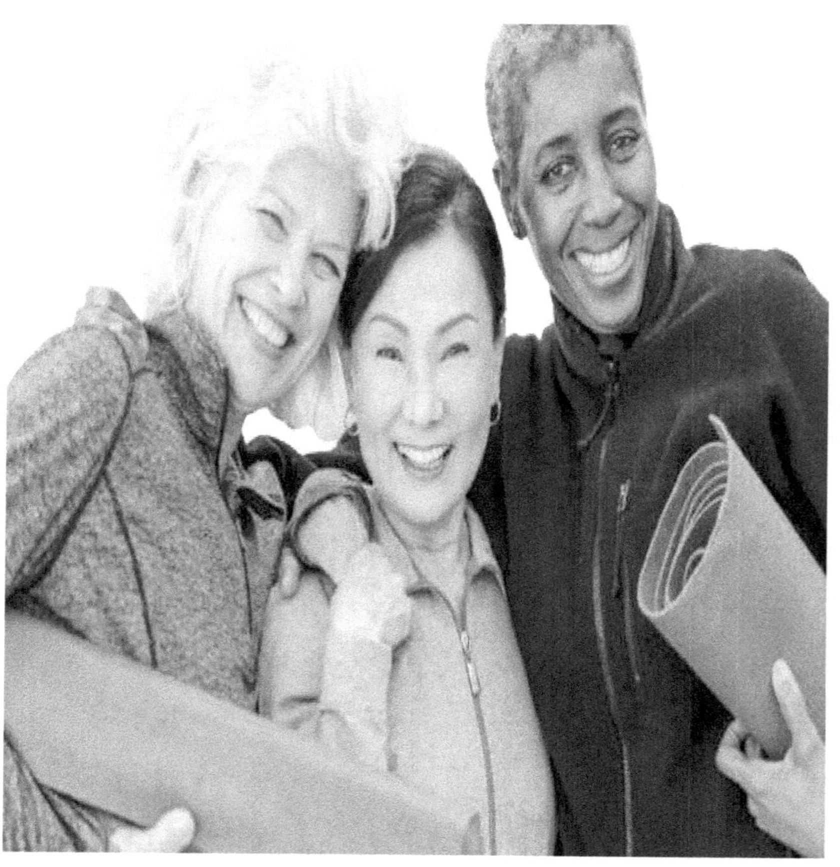

CHAPTER 6

Managing Complications and Coexisting Conditions for Congestive Heart Failure

Congestive heart failure (CHF) is a complex condition that can give rise to various complications and coexisting conditions. Effectively managing these additional health challenges is crucial for optimizing patient outcomes and enhancing their quality of life. In this comprehensive guide, we explore common complications and coexisting conditions associated with CHF and discuss strategies for their management.

1. Coronary Artery Disease (CAD):

Coronary artery disease often coexists with CHF and can further compromise heart function. Managing CAD involves strategies such as lifestyle modifications (e.g., a heart-healthy diet, regular exercise), medications to control blood pressure and cholesterol levels, and, in some cases, interventions such as percutaneous coronary intervention

(PCI) or coronary artery bypass grafting (CABG) to improve blood flow to the heart.

2. Arrhythmias:

Arrhythmias, including atrial fibrillation, are common in CHF and can exacerbate symptoms and increase the risk of complications. Treatment options include antiarrhythmic medications, electrical cardioversion, catheter ablation, and implantable devices (such as pacemakers or implantable cardioverter-defibrillators) to regulate heart rhythm and prevent life-threatening arrhythmias.

3. Hypertension:

Hypertension (high blood pressure) is a significant risk factor for the development and progression of CHF. Effective management involves lifestyle modifications, such as a low-sodium diet and regular exercise, as well as antihypertensive medications prescribed by a healthcare professional. Blood pressure monitoring and regular follow-up visits are crucial to ensure optimal control.

4. Diabetes:

Diabetes mellitus is commonly seen in individuals with CHF and can worsen heart function and increase the risk of complications. Managing diabetes requires a combination of lifestyle modifications (healthy diet, regular exercise), glucose monitoring, and medications (such as oral antidiabetic agents or insulin therapy) tailored to individual needs. Close coordination between healthcare providers specializing in cardiology and endocrinology is essential for comprehensive care.

5. Pulmonary Hypertension:

Pulmonary hypertension, characterized by increased blood pressure in the arteries of the lungs, often accompanies CHF. Treatment approaches may include medications to dilate blood vessels, diuretics to reduce fluid accumulation, and oxygen therapy. In severe cases, advanced therapies such as pulmonary artery vasodilators or lung transplantation may be considered.

6. Kidney Dysfunction:

Kidney dysfunction is both a cause and consequence of CHF and requires careful management to optimize heart and renal function. Treatment strategies involve controlling fluid and sodium intake, prescribing diuretics, and closely monitoring kidney function. In advanced cases, renal replacement therapies such as dialysis or kidney transplantation may be necessary.

7. Anemia:

Anemia is common in CHF and can exacerbate symptoms and reduce exercise capacity. Treatment may involve addressing underlying causes of anemia, such as iron deficiency, and, if necessary, prescribing medications to stimulate red blood cell production or providing blood transfusions.

8. Sleep-Disordered Breathing:

Conditions like sleep apnea can worsen heart function and increase the risk of cardiovascular events in individuals with CHF.

Managing sleep-disordered breathing involves continuous positive airway pressure (CPAP) therapy, weight management, and positional changes during sleep.

9. Psychological and Emotional Support:

Living with CHF and managing its complications can take a toll on an individual's psychological and emotional well-being. Supportive care, counseling, and involvement in support groups can help individuals cope with the challenges, reduce stress, and improve overall mental health.

10. Palliative and End-of-Life Care:

For individuals with advanced CHF who are not candidates for advanced interventions, palliative care focuses on symptom management, enhancing quality of life, and providing emotional support. Hospice care may be considered in the end stages of the disease, offering comfort and support for both the patient and their loved ones.

In conclusion, effectively managing complications and coexisting conditions in congestive heart failure is crucial for optimizing patient outcomes and enhancing their quality of life. A multidisciplinary approach involving healthcare providers from cardiology, nephrology, endocrinology, and other specialties is essential to provide comprehensive care tailored to individual needs. By addressing these challenges, we can improve the overall management of congestive heart failure and support individuals in their journey toward better health and well-being.

Arrhythmias and Heart Rhythm Disorders

Congestive heart failure (CHF) is often accompanied by arrhythmias and heart rhythm disorders, which can further complicate the condition and impact patient outcomes.

In this comprehensive guide, we delve into the intricacies of arrhythmias in the context of CHF, explore common types of heart rhythm disorders, and discuss strategies for their understanding, management, and restoration.

1. Arrhythmias in Congestive Heart Failure:

Arrhythmias refer to abnormal heart rhythms that can occur in individuals with CHF. These irregular rhythms can disrupt the efficient pumping of the heart, leading to symptoms such as palpitations, dizziness, shortness of breath, and fatigue. Common types of arrhythmias in CHF include:

a. Atrial Fibrillation (AF): AF is characterized by rapid and irregular electrical activity in the atria, leading to inefficient blood pumping. It is a prevalent arrhythmia in CHF and requires appropriate management to control heart rate and reduce the risk of blood clots.

b. Ventricular Arrhythmias: These arrhythmias originate in the ventricles and can be life-threatening. They include ventricular tachycardia (rapid heart rate) and ventricular fibrillation (chaotic electrical activity). Prompt intervention, such as defibrillation, is crucial for restoring normal heart rhythm.

c. Supraventricular Arrhythmias: These arrhythmias occur above the ventricles and can include conditions such as supraventricular tachycardia (SVT) or atrial flutter. Effective management involves controlling heart rate and, in some cases, restoring sinus rhythm.

2. Understanding Heart Rhythm Disorders:

Heart rhythm disorders encompass a broad range of conditions that affect the electrical system of the heart. In CHF, these disorders can arise due to structural abnormalities, impaired conduction pathways, electrolyte imbalances, or the presence of scar tissue from previous heart damage. Common heart rhythm disorders in CHF include:

a. Sinus Node Dysfunction: The sinus node, the heart's natural pacemaker, may malfunction, leading to slow heart rates (sinus bradycardia) or periods of no electrical activity (sinus arrest). This may result in symptoms such as dizziness, fainting, and fatigue.

b. Heart Block: Heart block refers to the interruption or delay in the electrical signals between the atria and ventricles. It can range from mild to severe and may require pacemaker implantation to regulate the heart's electrical conduction.

c. Long QT Syndrome: This inherited condition affects the heart's repolarization process, leading to a prolonged QT interval on the electrocardiogram (ECG). Prolonged QT intervals can predispose individuals to dangerous arrhythmias, including torsades de pointes.

3. Diagnosis and Evaluation:

Accurate diagnosis and evaluation of arrhythmias and heart rhythm disorders in CHF are crucial for effective management. This involves:

a. Electrocardiogram (ECG): An ECG records the electrical activity of the heart and can identify abnormal rhythms and conduction abnormalities.

b. Holter Monitoring: This portable device records the heart's electrical activity over a prolonged period (typically 24 to 48 hours), capturing intermittent arrhythmias that may not be detected during a standard ECG.

c. Electrophysiology Study (EPS): An EPS involves threading specialized catheters through blood vessels to the heart to assess its electrical system. It helps identify the specific location and mechanisms of arrhythmias and guides treatment decisions.

d. Echocardiogram: An echocardiogram assesses the heart's structure, function, and pumping capacity. It can provide valuable information about the underlying causes and severity of CHF.

4. Management of Arrhythmias and Heart Rhythm Disorders:

Effectively managing arrhythmias in the context of CHF requires a multifaceted approach, including:

a. Medications: Antiarrhythmic medications may be prescribed to control heart rhythm and rate. They can include beta-blockers, calcium channel blockers, and sodium channel blockers. These medications help stabilize electrical activity and reduce the risk of life-threatening arrhythmias.

b. Cardioversion: Cardioversion involves delivering a controlled electric shock to the heart to restore normal sinus rhythm. It can be performed as either electrical cardioversion (using a defibrillator) or pharmacological cardioversion (using medications).

c. Catheter Ablation: In this procedure, catheters are used to deliver energy (radiofrequency or cryotherapy) to the specific areas of the heart responsible for generating abnormal rhythms. It aims to eliminate the arrhythmia source and restore normal cardiac rhythm.

d. Pacemaker Implantation: Pacemakers are small electronic devices implanted under the skin that regulate the heart's electrical activity. They can be used to treat bradycardias, heart block, and certain types of arrhythmias.

e. Implantable Cardioverter-Defibrillator (ICD): ICDs are similar to pacemakers but can also deliver a shock to the heart to terminate life-threatening arrhythmias such as ventricular tachycardia or fibrillation.

5. Collaborative Care and Follow-Up:

Managing arrhythmias in the context of CHF requires a collaborative approach involving cardiologists, electrophysiologists, and other healthcare professionals.

Regular follow-up visits, adjustments to medication regimens, and lifestyle modifications may be necessary to ensure optimal management and minimize the risk of arrhythmia-related complications.

In conclusion, arrhythmias and heart rhythm disorders significantly impact the management and prognosis of congestive heart failure. By understanding the types of arrhythmias, their underlying causes, and employing a comprehensive approach to diagnosis and treatment, healthcare professionals can effectively manage these conditions and improve patient outcomes. With advancements in diagnostic techniques, interventional procedures, and implantable devices, there is an increasing range of options available to restore and regulate cardiac rhythm, thereby enhancing the quality of life for individuals with CHF.

Hypertension and High Blood Pressure

Hypertension, also known as high blood pressure, is a significant risk factor for the development and progression of congestive heart failure (CHF). The coexistence of hypertension and CHF poses unique challenges for patients and healthcare providers.

In this comprehensive guide, we explore the intricacies of hypertension in the context of CHF, its impact on cardiac function, and strategies for understanding, managing, and controlling this silent threat.

1. The Link between Hypertension and Congestive Heart Failure:

Hypertension refers to chronically elevated blood pressure, and it can lead to damage in the blood vessels, heart, and other organs. Over time, uncontrolled hypertension places excessive strain on the heart, resulting in structural changes, impaired heart function, and ultimately contributing to the development of CHF. Additionally, hypertension can worsen existing CHF by increasing fluid retention and causing further damage to the heart muscle.

2. Understanding Hypertension in Congestive Heart Failure:

a. Systolic vs. Diastolic Hypertension: Systolic hypertension occurs when the top number of the blood pressure reading is consistently elevated, indicating increased pressure when the heart contracts.

Diastolic hypertension refers to a consistently elevated bottom number, indicating increased pressure when the heart is at rest. Both types can contribute to CHF.

b. Pulmonary Hypertension: Hypertension can also affect the pulmonary arteries, leading to pulmonary hypertension. Increased pressure in the lungs makes it more challenging for the heart to pump blood efficiently, exacerbating the symptoms and complications of CHF.

3. Diagnosis and Evaluation:

Accurate diagnosis and evaluation of hypertension in the context of CHF are crucial for optimal management. This involves:

a. Blood Pressure Measurement: Regular monitoring of blood pressure, both in a healthcare setting and at home, is essential to identify and track hypertension. Ambulatory blood pressure monitoring (ABPM) may be used to assess blood pressure patterns over a 24-hour period.

b. Diagnostic Tests: Additional tests, such as echocardiography, electrocardiogram (ECG), and laboratory evaluations, may be performed to assess heart function, identify any underlying causes of hypertension, and determine the presence of associated conditions such as kidney disease or diabetes.

4. Management and Control of Hypertension in CHF:
Managing hypertension in the context of CHF involves a comprehensive approach that includes:

a. Lifestyle Modifications: Encouraging lifestyle changes is crucial in the management of hypertension. This can include adopting a heart-healthy diet (low in sodium and saturated fats, rich in fruits, vegetables, and whole grains), regular physical activity, weight management, stress reduction techniques, and moderation in alcohol consumption.

b. Medications: Antihypertensive medications are often prescribed to control blood pressure in CHF patients.

These may include angiotensin-converting enzyme (ACE) inhibitors, angiotensin receptor blockers (ARBs), beta-blockers, diuretics, calcium channel blockers, or a combination of these medications. The choice of medication depends on the individual's specific needs and any underlying conditions.

c. Salt Restriction: Limiting sodium intake is vital for managing fluid retention and controlling blood pressure. Healthcare providers may recommend a specific sodium restriction and provide guidance on reading food labels, cooking methods, and alternatives to high-sodium seasonings.

d. Regular Monitoring and Follow-Up: Close monitoring of blood pressure and regular follow-up visits with healthcare providers are necessary to ensure blood pressure control, assess medication effectiveness, and make any necessary adjustments to the treatment plan.

5. Collaborative Care:

Effective management of hypertension in CHF requires a collaborative approach involving healthcare providers specializing in cardiology, primary care, and other relevant specialties. Regular communication, shared decision-making, and patient education are key to empowering individuals with CHF to actively participate in their care and maintain optimal blood pressure control.

In conclusion, hypertension and high blood pressure significantly impact the development, progression, and management of congestive heart failure. By understanding the link between hypertension and CHF, implementing lifestyle modifications, prescribing appropriate medications, and closely monitoring blood pressure, healthcare providers can help patients achieve optimal blood pressure control, reduce the risk of complications, and improve overall outcomes in the management of both conditions. Empowering patients with knowledge and support is vital in promoting self-management and fostering a collaborative approach to care.

Coronary Artery Disease (CAD)

Coronary Artery Disease (CAD) and Congestive Heart Failure (CHF) are two interconnected cardiovascular conditions that often coexist, amplifying the challenges faced by patients and healthcare providers. In this comprehensive guide, we explore the intricate relationship between CAD and CHF, their impact on each other, diagnostic considerations, treatment approaches, and strategies for managing these conditions simultaneously.

1. Understanding the Intersection of CAD and CHF:

a. Shared Pathophysiology: CAD refers to the narrowing or blockage of the coronary arteries, impairing blood flow to the heart muscle. CHF, on the other hand, is characterized by the heart's inability to pump blood effectively. CAD can be a primary cause of CHF or contribute to its development by reducing blood supply to the heart and causing myocardial damage.

b. Impact on Cardiac Function: CAD can weaken the heart muscle over time, leading to or exacerbating CHF.

The impaired blood flow caused by CAD can result in myocardial infarction (heart attack), further compromising cardiac function and worsening CHF symptoms.

2. Diagnostic Considerations:

Accurate diagnosis of CAD and CHF in combination requires a comprehensive evaluation, which may include:

a. Medical History: Understanding a patient's medical history, including any previous heart conditions, risk factors, and prior interventions, provides important insights for diagnosis and management.

b. Symptom Assessment: Patients with CAD and CHF may experience symptoms such as chest pain, shortness of breath, fatigue, and fluid retention. Evaluating the nature, severity, and progression of these symptoms helps guide diagnosis and treatment.

c. Diagnostic Tests: Diagnostic tests such as electrocardiogram (ECG), echocardiography, stress testing, cardiac catheterization, and coronary angiography may be performed to assess cardiac function, detect CAD-related blockages, and determine the extent of coronary artery involvement.

3. Treatment Approaches for CAD in CHF:

Managing CAD in the context of CHF requires a comprehensive treatment approach that addresses both conditions:

a. Medications: Medications for CAD and CHF may overlap, including antiplatelet agents (such as aspirin), beta-blockers, ACE inhibitors or angiotensin receptor blockers (ARBs), diuretics, and cholesterol-lowering drugs (statins). The choice of medications depends on the patient's specific needs, symptomatology, and underlying conditions.

b. Revascularization Procedures: In cases where CAD is severe and significantly impacts cardiac function, revascularization procedures such as percutaneous coronary intervention (PCI) with stent placement or coronary artery bypass grafting (CABG) may be essential to restore blood flow to the heart.

c. Cardiac Rehabilitation: Cardiac rehabilitation programs can help patients with CAD and CHF improve their physical fitness, manage symptoms, and adopt heart-healthy lifestyle modifications.

4. Lifestyle Modifications and Self-Care:

Promoting healthy lifestyle habits is crucial in managing CAD and CHF:

a. Heart-Healthy Diet: Emphasize a balanced diet rich in fruits, vegetables, whole grains, lean proteins, and low in saturated fats, cholesterol, and sodium. Encourage portion control and nutritional counseling.

b. Regular Physical Activity: Encourage patients to engage in regular exercise as recommended by healthcare providers, taking into account their individual capabilities and limitations. Physical activity helps strengthen the heart, improve circulation, and manage weight.

c. Smoking Cessation: Educate patients about the risks of smoking and support them in quitting. Smoking cessation is vital in reducing further damage to the heart and improving overall cardiovascular health.

d. Weight Management: Maintaining a healthy weight can alleviate strain on the heart and improve overall cardiac function. Encourage patients to achieve and maintain a healthy body weight through a combination of diet and exercise.

5. Ongoing Monitoring and Follow-up:

Regular monitoring and follow-up are essential to assess treatment efficacy, manage symptoms, and identify any changes or complications.

Patients with CAD and CHF may require periodic cardiac evaluations, imaging studies, blood tests, and medication adjustments to optimize their management.

In conclusion, the coexistence of CAD and CHF presents a complex challenge in cardiovascular care. By understanding the interplay between these conditions, healthcare providers can tailor treatment plans that address both CAD and CHF, improve cardiac function, alleviate symptoms, and enhance overall quality of life for patients. Empowering individuals with knowledge about their conditions, promoting healthy lifestyle modifications, and ensuring consistent medical follow-up are essential components of managing CAD and CHF simultaneously.

Diabetes and Heart Failure in Congestive Heart Failure (CHF): A Complex Interplay, Implications, and Management Strategies

The coexistence of diabetes and congestive heart failure (CHF) creates a challenging clinical scenario, as both conditions influence each other and significantly impact patient outcomes. In this comprehensive guide, we explore the intricate relationship between diabetes, CHF, their underlying mechanisms, diagnostic considerations, treatment approaches, and strategies for managing these conditions concurrently.

1. Understanding the Interplay between Diabetes and CHF:

a. Shared Pathophysiology: Diabetes and CHF share common underlying mechanisms, including chronic inflammation, oxidative stress, endothelial dysfunction, and impaired insulin signaling. These processes contribute to the development and progression of both conditions.

b. Bidirectional Relationship: Diabetes is a significant risk factor for developing CHF, and patients with CHF are more likely to have diabetes compared to the general population. The presence of diabetes in CHF patients is associated with worse outcomes, increased hospitalizations, and higher mortality rates.

2. Diagnostic Considerations:

Accurate diagnosis and evaluation of diabetes and CHF in combination require a comprehensive approach:

a. Medical History: Assessing a patient's medical history, including any history of diabetes, CHF-related symptoms, medication use, and glycemic control, helps guide diagnosis and management.

b. Diagnostic Tests: Diagnostic tests such as blood glucose measurement, glycated hemoglobin (HbA1c) testing, echocardiography, and cardiac imaging studies are essential in assessing diabetes control, cardiac function, and identifying any structural abnormalities associated with CHF.

3. Treatment Approaches for Diabetes and CHF:

Managing diabetes and CHF concurrently involves a comprehensive treatment strategy that addresses both conditions:

a. Glycemic Control: Achieving and maintaining optimal blood glucose levels is essential in diabetes management. Lifestyle modifications, oral antidiabetic medications, and insulin therapy may be employed based on individual patient needs.

b. Medications for CHF: Medications commonly used for CHF, such as beta-blockers, angiotensin-converting enzyme (ACE) inhibitors or angiotensin receptor blockers (ARBs), and diuretics, should be prescribed with careful consideration of their effects on glycemic control.

c. Cardiovascular Risk Reduction: Aggressive management of cardiovascular risk factors, including hypertension, dyslipidemia, and smoking cessation, is crucial in both diabetes and CHF management.

4. Lifestyle Modifications and Self-Care:

Promoting healthy lifestyle habits is essential in managing diabetes and CHF:

a. Balanced Diet: Encourage a heart-healthy diet rich in fruits, vegetables, whole grains, lean proteins, and low in saturated fats, cholesterol, and sodium. Emphasize portion control and regular meal timing.

b. Regular Physical Activity: Encourage patients to engage in regular exercise as recommended by healthcare providers. Physical activity helps improve insulin sensitivity, cardiovascular fitness, and overall well-being.

c. Medication Adherence: Encourage adherence to prescribed medications for both diabetes and CHF.

Medications for diabetes management, such as antidiabetic agents and insulin, should be taken as directed.

d. Blood Pressure and Cholesterol Management: Ensure optimal control of blood pressure and cholesterol levels through medication, lifestyle modifications, and regular monitoring.

5. Ongoing Monitoring and Collaborative Care:

Regular monitoring and collaborative care are vital in managing diabetes and CHF:

a. Regular Medical Follow-up: Schedule regular follow-up appointments to assess glycemic control, cardiac function, medication adjustments, and address any emerging concerns.

b. Team-based Approach: Collaborate with a multidisciplinary team, including endocrinologists, cardiologists, primary care physicians, and diabetes educators, to provide comprehensive care and ensure optimal management of both conditions.

c. Patient Education: Educate patients about the importance of self-monitoring of blood glucose levels, recognizing CHF-related symptoms, and adhering to prescribed medications and lifestyle modifications.

In conclusion, the intersection of diabetes and CHF presents complex challenges in patient management. By understanding the interplay between these conditions, healthcare providers can develop tailored treatment plans that address both diabetes and CHF, optimize glycemic control, improve cardiac function, reduce cardiovascular risk, and enhance overall quality of life. Empowering patients with knowledge, promoting healthy lifestyle modifications, and ensuring regular medical follow-up are essential components of managing diabetes and CHF simultaneously.

CHAPTER 7

Emotional and Mental Well-being in Congestive Heart Failure (CHF): Understanding the Importance, Impact, and Strategies for Support

Congestive Heart Failure (CHF) not only affects the physical health of individuals but also has a significant impact on their emotional and mental well-being. The emotional and psychological aspects of living with CHF should be acknowledged and addressed as part of a comprehensive care approach. In this comprehensive guide, we explore the importance of emotional and mental well-being in CHF, the challenges individuals may face, and strategies for supporting their mental health.

1. Understanding the Importance of Emotional and Mental Well-being in CHF:

a. Psychological Impact: CHF can lead to emotional distress, anxiety, depression, and reduced quality of life. The experience of managing a chronic condition, dealing with physical limitations, and facing uncertainties about the future can take a toll on mental well-being.

b. Impact on Physical Health: Emotional and mental well-being can influence the management of CHF. Poor mental health may lead to non-adherence to medication and treatment plans, unhealthy lifestyle choices, and increased stress, which can exacerbate CHF symptoms and increase the risk of hospitalizations.

2. Challenges Faced by Individuals with CHF:

a. Anxiety and Worry: Living with CHF may lead to heightened anxiety and worry about disease progression, symptoms, and potential complications. The fear of breathlessness, fatigue, and limitations in daily activities can cause distress.

b. Depression and Emotional Distress: CHF can contribute to feelings of sadness, hopelessness, and a loss of interest in previously enjoyed activities. Individuals may experience a sense of isolation, difficulty coping with changes in physical abilities, and frustration related to the impact of CHF on their lifestyle.

c. Lifestyle Adjustments: Adapting to lifestyle changes, such as dietary modifications, fluid restrictions, medication schedules, and physical activity limitations, can be emotionally challenging. It may require support and adjustment to maintain a positive outlook and engage in self-care practices effectively.

3. Strategies for Supporting Emotional and Mental Well-being:

a. Education and Counseling: Providing individuals with CHF and their families with information about the condition, its management, and potential emotional challenges can empower them to cope better.

Counseling and support groups can offer a safe space for individuals to express their feelings, share experiences, and gain coping strategies.

b. Psychosocial Support: Encourage individuals with CHF to seek social support from family, friends, or support networks. Engaging in activities that promote social interaction and maintaining connections can help reduce feelings of isolation.

c. Cognitive-Behavioral Therapy (CBT): CBT techniques, including relaxation exercises, cognitive restructuring, and stress management strategies, can help individuals develop effective coping mechanisms, challenge negative thoughts, and reduce anxiety or depression symptoms.

d. Self-Care and Stress Reduction: Encourage individuals with CHF to prioritize self-care activities that promote relaxation and stress reduction, such as mindfulness meditation, deep breathing exercises, adequate sleep, and engaging in hobbies or activities they enjoy.

e. Collaboration with Mental Health Professionals: Collaborate with mental health professionals, such as psychologists or psychiatrists, to provide specialized support for individuals with CHF who may require additional intervention or medication management for mental health concerns.

f. Caregiver Support: Acknowledge the vital role of caregivers and provide support and resources to help them manage their own emotional well-being. Caregivers may experience stress, fatigue, and emotional exhaustion, and offering them assistance and respite care can alleviate their burden.

4. Integration of Mental Health Support into Care Plans:

Incorporate routine assessments of emotional and mental well-being into the overall care plan for individuals with CHF.

Regular screenings for depression, anxiety, and other mental health concerns can help identify individuals who may require additional support or referral to mental health professionals.

In conclusion, recognizing the importance of emotional and mental well-being in individuals with CHF is essential for comprehensive care. By addressing the emotional and psychological aspects of CHF, healthcare providers can improve quality of life, enhance treatment adherence, and promote better overall outcomes. Implementing strategies for support, collaboration with mental health professionals, and promoting self-care practices can contribute to the holistic management of individuals with CHF and their mental well-being.

Coping with the Emotional Impact of Congestive Heart Failure (CHF)

Living with Congestive Heart Failure (CHF) can be emotionally challenging, as it brings about various physical, lifestyle, and emotional changes. Coping with the emotional impact of CHF is crucial for maintaining psychological well-being and improving overall quality of life. In this comprehensive guide, we explore strategies and techniques to help individuals effectively cope with the emotional challenges associated with CHF.

1. Acknowledge and Validate Emotions:

Recognize that it is normal to experience a range of emotions when living with CHF. Allow yourself to acknowledge and accept these emotions, whether it's fear, frustration, sadness, or anxiety. Validating your emotions can help you navigate them in a healthier way.

2. Seek Emotional Support:

a. Open Communication: Share your feelings and concerns with your loved ones, friends, or a support group. Talking about your emotions can provide relief and foster understanding and support.

b. Professional Counseling: Consider seeking the help of a mental health professional, such as a psychologist or counselor, who can provide specialized guidance and support in managing the emotional impact of CHF.

c. Support Groups: Joining a support group specifically tailored for individuals with CHF can provide a sense of community and understanding. Hearing others' experiences and sharing your own can help alleviate feelings of isolation and offer practical coping strategies.

3. Educate Yourself:

Learn as much as you can about CHF, its management, and self-care strategies.

Understanding your condition can empower you to make informed decisions, alleviate anxiety, and enhance your sense of control over your health.

4. Develop Coping Mechanisms:

a. Stress Management Techniques: Practice relaxation techniques such as deep breathing exercises, meditation, mindfulness, or progressive muscle relaxation. These techniques can help reduce stress levels and promote a sense of calmness.

b. Cognitive-Behavioral Strategies: Challenge negative thoughts and cognitive distortions by reframing them with more positive and realistic perspectives. Engage in positive self-talk and focus on your strengths and achievements.

c. Goal Setting: Set achievable goals that align with your capabilities and values. Breaking larger tasks into smaller, manageable steps can bring a sense of accomplishment and motivation.

5. Engage in Self-Care:

a. Prioritize Physical Health: Adhere to your prescribed medication regimen, maintain a healthy diet, and engage in regular physical activity as recommended by your healthcare provider. Physical well-being can positively impact your emotional state.

b. Establish a Routine: Create a structured routine that includes regular sleep patterns, meal times, medication schedules, and self-care activities. A routine can provide a sense of stability and control amidst the challenges of CHF.

c. Engage in Enjoyable Activities: Make time for hobbies, interests, and activities that bring you joy and relaxation. Engaging in pleasurable activities can help uplift your mood and provide a sense of fulfillment.

6. Practice Acceptance and Adaptation:

Accepting and adapting to the changes brought about by CHF can be a transformative process.

Focus on what you can control and adjust your expectations and goals accordingly. Embrace self-compassion and give yourself permission to make necessary lifestyle adjustments.

7. Communicate with Your Healthcare Team:

Keep the lines of communication with your healthcare team open and honest. Regularly discuss your emotional well-being, any concerns, or challenges you may be facing. They can provide guidance, offer additional resources, or make appropriate referrals to mental health professionals if needed.

In conclusion, coping with the emotional impact of CHF requires a multifaceted approach that combines self-awareness, emotional support, self-care practices, and effective communication with healthcare providers. By implementing these strategies, individuals can build resilience, improve their emotional well-being, and navigate the challenges of CHF with greater strength and positivity. Remember, you are not alone in this journey, and there is support available to help you cope and thrive.

Supportive Resources and Counseling

Living with Congestive Heart Failure (CHF) can present unique challenges, both physically and emotionally. To support individuals with CHF in managing their condition and promoting overall well-being, various supportive resources and counseling services are available. In this comprehensive guide, we explore the different types of resources and counseling options that can provide valuable support and guidance to individuals with CHF.

1. Support Groups:

Support groups specifically tailored for individuals with CHF can offer a sense of community, understanding, and shared experiences. These groups typically provide a safe space for individuals to discuss their concerns, emotions, and challenges related to CHF. Support groups can be in-person or online, allowing individuals to connect with others who are facing similar situations. Sharing experiences, coping strategies, and receiving emotional support from peers can significantly benefit individuals with CHF.

2. Educational Programs:

Educational programs and classes focused on CHF management can provide valuable information, skills, and self-care strategies. These programs often cover topics such as medication management, dietary guidelines, physical activity recommendations, symptom recognition, and lifestyle modifications. Participating in educational programs can empower individuals with CHF to take an active role in their healthcare, make informed decisions, and enhance their overall well-being.

3. Individual Counseling:

Individual counseling or therapy sessions with mental health professionals, such as psychologists or licensed counselors, can be highly beneficial for individuals with CHF. These sessions offer a safe and confidential environment to discuss emotional concerns, anxiety, depression, and coping strategies. Mental health professionals can provide guidance, tools, and evidence-based therapeutic techniques to help individuals manage the emotional impact of CHF effectively.

They can also assist in developing healthy coping mechanisms, addressing self-esteem issues, and improving overall mental well-being.

4. Caregiver Support:

Congestive Heart Failure not only affects individuals with the condition but also their caregivers. Caregivers often experience emotional distress, stress, and burnout while providing care and support to their loved ones. Caregiver support groups, counseling services, or respite care programs can provide valuable resources and assistance to caregivers. These resources can help caregivers navigate the challenges, develop self-care strategies, and provide emotional support to maintain their own well-being while caring for someone with CHF.

5. Palliative Care and Hospice Services:

In advanced stages of CHF or for individuals with severe symptoms, palliative care or hospice services may be considered. These specialized services focus on providing comfort, pain management, and emotional support for individuals with advanced CHF and their families. Palliative care teams collaborate with healthcare professionals, including physicians, nurses, social workers, and counselors, to ensure holistic care and support during end-of-life stages.

6. Online Resources and Digital Apps:

There is a wide range of online resources and digital applications available that provide educational materials, self-help tools, symptom trackers, and support forums for individuals with CHF. These resources can be accessed conveniently from the comfort of one's home, offering information, tips, and interactive features to support CHF management and emotional well-being.

7. Collaborative Care Planning:

Collaborative care planning involves a multidisciplinary team approach where healthcare professionals, including cardiologists, nurses, social workers, and mental health professionals, work together to develop an individualized care plan for individuals with CHF. This integrated approach ensures that emotional well-being is considered along with medical management.

The team can provide ongoing support, monitor progress, and make appropriate referrals to counseling services or supportive resources when needed.

In conclusion, supportive resources and counseling services play a vital role in promoting emotional well-being, providing education, and offering guidance for individuals with CHF and their caregivers. Engaging in support groups, seeking individual counseling, accessing educational programs, and utilizing online resources can help individuals better cope with the emotional impact of CHF and enhance their overall quality of life. Remember, reaching out for support is a sign of strength, and these resources are designed to assist and empower you on your CHF journey.

CHAPTER 8

Preventive Measures and Lifestyle Tips

Prevention plays a crucial role in managing and reducing the risk of congestive heart failure (CHF). By adopting a heart-healthy lifestyle and implementing preventive measures, individuals can enhance their overall cardiovascular health and reduce the likelihood of developing CHF. In this comprehensive guide, we explore a range of preventive measures and lifestyle tips that can contribute to maintaining a healthy heart and minimizing the risk of CHF.

1. Healthy Diet:

a. Balanced Nutrition: Follow a well-balanced diet that includes a variety of fruits, vegetables, whole grains, lean proteins, and healthy fats. Limit the intake of processed foods, saturated fats, trans fats, cholesterol, sodium, and added sugars.

b. Sodium Restriction: Monitor and reduce sodium intake, as excessive sodium consumption can contribute to fluid retention and worsen CHF symptoms. Aim to limit sodium to less than 2,300 milligrams (mg) per day or as recommended by your healthcare provider.

c. Fluid Intake: Follow any fluid restriction guidelines provided by your healthcare team. Monitoring and moderating fluid intake can help manage fluid buildup and reduce strain on the heart.

d. Consult with a Registered Dietitian: Consider consulting with a registered dietitian who specializes in cardiovascular health. They can provide personalized dietary recommendations and support to help you make sustainable and heart-healthy food choices.

2. Regular Physical Activity:

a. Consult with Your Healthcare Provider: Before starting or modifying an exercise routine, consult with your healthcare provider to determine the appropriate level of physical activity for your condition. They can provide guidelines tailored to your needs and capabilities.

b. Aerobic Exercise: Engage in regular aerobic exercises, such as brisk walking, cycling, swimming, or dancing. According to the American Heart Association, you should strive to do at least 150 minutes of moderate-intensity aerobic activity or 75 minutes of vigorous-intensity aerobic activity per week.

c. Strength Training: Incorporate strength training exercises into your routine to improve muscle strength and endurance. Work with a certified fitness professional or physical therapist to develop a safe and effective strength training program.

d. Listen to Your Body: Pay attention to your body's signals during exercise. If you experience chest pain, severe shortness of breath, dizziness, or lightheadedness, stop exercising and seek medical attention.

3. Tobacco and Alcohol:

a. Quit Smoking: If you smoke, quitting is one of the most significant steps you can take to improve your heart health. Seek support from healthcare professionals, smoking cessation programs, or support groups to assist you in the quitting process.

b. Limit Alcohol Consumption: Moderate alcohol consumption (up to one drink per day for women and up to two drinks per day for men) may be acceptable for some individuals. However, excessive alcohol intake can contribute to heart problems. Consult with your healthcare provider to determine if alcohol consumption is appropriate for your situation.

4. Medication Adherence:

a. Follow Prescribed Medications: Take your medications as prescribed by your healthcare provider. Medications such as ACE inhibitors, beta-blockers, diuretics, and others are commonly prescribed for CHF management and prevention.

Adhering to the prescribed regimen can help control symptoms, manage blood pressure, and reduce the risk of complications.

b. Regular Medication Review: Periodically review your medications with your healthcare provider to ensure they are still appropriate for your condition and to address any potential side effects or interactions.

5. Stress Management:

a. Relaxation Techniques: Practice stress management techniques such as deep breathing exercises, meditation, yoga, or tai chi to help reduce stress and promote relaxation.

b. Engage in Hobbies and Activities: Find activities that bring you joy and help you unwind. Engaging in hobbies, spending time with loved ones, or participating in activities you enjoy can help alleviate stress and improve overall well-being.

6. Regular Medical Check-ups:

a. Routine Follow-up: Schedule regular follow-up appointments with your healthcare provider to monitor your heart health, review your condition, adjust medications if necessary, and discuss any concerns or symptoms you may be experiencing.

b. Screenings and Vaccinations: Stay up to date with recommended health screenings, such as blood pressure checks, cholesterol screenings, and vaccinations (including flu and pneumonia vaccines). These preventive measures can help identify and manage any potential risk factors.

7. Sleep Hygiene:

a. Establish a Sleep Routine: Aim for seven to eight hours of quality sleep per night.

Establish a consistent sleep schedule, create a conducive sleep environment, and adopt healthy sleep hygiene practices.

b. Address Sleep Apnea: If you have symptoms of sleep apnea, such as loud snoring, interrupted breathing during sleep, or excessive daytime sleepiness, discuss these concerns with your healthcare provider. Treating sleep apnea can improve heart health and overall well-being.

8. Maintain a Healthy Weight:

a. Body Weight Management: Maintain a healthy weight range through a combination of regular physical activity and a balanced diet. Achieving and maintaining a healthy weight can help reduce strain on the heart and improve overall cardiovascular health.

b. Consult with a Healthcare Professional: If you need guidance on weight management, consult with a registered dietitian or healthcare provider who can provide personalized recommendations based on your specific needs and goals.

In conclusion, adopting preventive measures and implementing lifestyle changes are crucial in managing and reducing the risk of congestive heart failure.

By embracing a healthy diet, engaging in regular physical activity, avoiding tobacco and excessive alcohol consumption, adhering to medications, managing stress, attending regular medical check-ups, prioritizing sleep, and maintaining a healthy weight, you can promote heart health and enhance your overall well-being. Remember to consult with your healthcare provider for personalized advice and guidance tailored to your individual needs and medical condition.

Promoting Heart-Healthy Habits for Congestive Heart Failure (CHF)

In congestive heart failure (CHF), adopting heart-healthy habits plays a crucial role in managing the condition, improving cardiovascular wellness, and enhancing overall quality of life.

By incorporating these comprehensive and detailed strategies into daily routines, individuals can optimize heart health and promote well-being.

Let's explore a range of effective habits to support individuals with CHF in their journey toward a heart-healthy lifestyle.

1. Balanced and Nutritious Diet:

- Consume a range of nutrient-dense foods, including fruits, vegetables, whole grains, lean proteins, and healthy fats.

- Reduce the intake of saturated fats, trans fats, cholesterol, sodium, and added sugars.

- Opt for low-sodium alternatives and use herbs and spices to flavor meals instead of salt.

- Consider working with a registered dietitian to develop a personalized eating plan tailored to your specific needs and preferences.

2. Regular Physical Activity:

- Engage in regular aerobic exercises such as walking, swimming, cycling, or dancing. According to the American Heart Association, you should strive to do at least 150 minutes of moderate-intensity aerobic activity or 75 minutes of vigorous-intensity aerobic activity per week.

- Improve muscle strength and endurance by including strength training workouts. Work with a certified fitness professional or physical therapist to develop a safe and effective strength training program.

- Remember to consult with your healthcare provider before starting or modifying an exercise routine to ensure it is appropriate for your condition.

3. Medication Adherence:

- Follow your prescribed medications as directed by your healthcare provider. Medications commonly prescribed for CHF include ACE inhibitors, beta-blockers, diuretics, and others.

- Adhering to the prescribed regimen is crucial for managing symptoms, controlling blood pressure, and reducing the risk of complications.

- Keep a record of your medications, their dosages, and any specific instructions. Use pill organizers or smartphone apps to help you stay organized and ensure you take your medications as scheduled.

- Regularly communicate with your healthcare provider about any concerns or side effects related to your medications.

4. Smoking Cessation:

- Quit smoking if you are a smoker. Smoking is a significant risk factor for heart disease and can worsen CHF symptoms. Seek support from healthcare professionals, smoking cessation programs, or support groups to assist you in quitting.

- Avoid exposure to secondhand smoke, as it can also contribute to heart problems.

5. Stress Management:

- Use stress management techniques such as deep breathing exercises, meditation, yoga, or engaging in hobbies and activities you enjoy.

- Prioritize self-care and relaxation, and make time for activities that promote a sense of calm and well-being.

- Consider seeking professional help from mental health professionals if you experience significant stress or anxiety related to your condition.

6. Adequate Sleep:

- Each night, try to get seven to eight hours of restful sleep. Establish a consistent sleep routine and create a comfortable sleep environment.

- Address any sleep disturbances or conditions such as sleep apnea by consulting with your healthcare provider. Treating sleep-related issues can have a positive impact on your heart health.

7. Limit Alcohol Consumption:

- If you decide to consume alcohol, do so moderately. The American Heart Association recommends limiting alcohol intake to up to one drink per day for women and up to two drinks per day for men.

- Excessive alcohol consumption can contribute to heart problems and should be avoided.

8. Regular Medical Check-ups and Monitoring:

- Schedule regular follow-up appointments with your healthcare provider to monitor your heart health, review your condition, and adjust your treatment plan if necessary.

- Stay up to date with recommended health screenings, such as blood pressure checks, cholesterol screenings, and other tests to assess your cardiovascular health.

9. Support Network and Emotional Well-being:

- Surround yourself with a supportive network of family, friends, and healthcare professionals who can provide encouragement and understanding.
- Seek emotional support when needed, such as joining support groups, counseling, or therapy. Emotional well-being is an integral part of managing CHF effectively.

10. Education and Self-Management:

- Educate yourself about CHF, its symptoms, treatment options, and self-management strategies. Understanding your condition empowers you to make informed decisions and actively participate in your care.

- Keep a journal to track your symptoms, medications, diet, exercise, and overall well-being. This can help you identify patterns, triggers, and progress in managing your condition.

Remember, it's necessary to consult with your healthcare provider before making any significant changes to your lifestyle or treatment plan. They can provide personalized guidance and support tailored to your specific needs and condition.

By implementing these heart-healthy habits and adopting a proactive approach to self-care, you can optimize your heart health and enhance your overall well-being while living with congestive heart failure.

Reducing Risk Factors for Heart Failure

Reducing risk factors for heart failure is essential in preventing or managing this condition. By adopting a comprehensive approach to cardiovascular health, individuals can minimize their risk and promote overall well-being. Let's explore comprehensive and detailed strategies to reduce risk factors for heart failure:

1. Maintain a Healthy Weight:

- By eating a balanced diet and getting regular exercise, you can achieve a healthy body weight.

- Incorporate nutrient-rich foods, such as fruits, vegetables, whole grains, lean proteins, and healthy fats, while limiting the intake of saturated fats, trans fats, cholesterol, sodium, and added sugars.

- Consult with a registered dietitian for personalized guidance on weight management and healthy eating habits.

2. Engage in Regular Physical Activity:

- Include regular exercise in your routine, aiming for at least 150 minutes of moderate-intensity aerobic activity or 75 minutes of vigorous-intensity aerobic activity per week.

- Choose activities you enjoy, such as walking, swimming, cycling, or dancing, and gradually increase the intensity and duration of your workouts.

- Consider strength training exercises to improve muscle strength and endurance, which can further support heart health.

- Consult with your healthcare provider before starting or modifying an exercise program to ensure it is suitable for your condition.

3. Control Blood Pressure:

- Monitor and manage your blood pressure regularly, aiming for a target of less than 130/80 mmHg, or as recommended by your healthcare provider.

- Implement lifestyle modifications such as maintaining a healthy weight, reducing sodium intake, adopting a heart-healthy diet, limiting alcohol consumption, and engaging in regular physical activity.

- If needed, your healthcare provider may prescribe medication to help control blood pressure.

Take medications as prescribed and attend regular check-ups to monitor your blood pressure.

4. Manage Cholesterol Levels:

- Follow a heart-healthy diet low in saturated and trans fats, cholesterol, and dietary cholesterol.

- Increase consumption of high-fiber foods, such as fruits, vegetables, whole grains, and legumes.

- Consider medications, such as statins, if lifestyle modifications alone are not sufficient to control cholesterol levels. Work with your healthcare provider to determine the most appropriate treatment plan for your condition.

5. Control Diabetes:

- Maintain good glycemic control if you have diabetes, as uncontrolled diabetes can increase the risk of heart failure.

- Monitor blood glucose levels regularly, follow a balanced diet, engage in regular physical activity, and take medications as prescribed by your healthcare provider.

- Work with a healthcare team, including a registered dietitian and diabetes educator, to manage your diabetes effectively.

6. Avoid Tobacco Smoke:

- Quit smoking if you are a smoker. Smoking damages blood vessels, increases blood pressure, and significantly raises the risk of heart disease and heart failure.

- Avoid exposure to secondhand smoke, as it can also be harmful to your cardiovascular health.

7. Limit Alcohol Consumption:

- If you decide to consume alcohol, do so moderately. The American Heart Association recommends limiting alcohol intake to up to one drink per day for women and up to two drinks per day for men.

- Drinking too much alcohol can raise blood pressure and cause heart issues.

8. Manage Stress:

- Adopt stress management techniques such as deep breathing exercises, meditation, yoga, or engaging in hobbies and activities that promote relaxation.
- Practice good time management, set realistic goals, and establish a healthy work-life balance.

- Seek support from loved ones, join support groups, or consider counseling or therapy to cope with stress effectively.

9. Get Regular Check-ups:

- Schedule regular check-ups with your healthcare provider to monitor your cardiovascular health, assess risk factors, and detect any potential issues early on.

- Follow recommended health screenings, including blood pressure checks, cholesterol screenings, diabetes screenings, and other relevant tests.

10. Stay Informed and Educated:

- Stay informed about heart health, cardiovascular risk factors, and the latest research in the field.

- Educate yourself about your personal risk factors, family history, and ways to manage and reduce those risks.

- Engage in shared decision-making with your healthcare provider to develop a personalized plan that suits your specific needs and goals.

By adopting these comprehensive strategies to reduce risk factors for heart failure, individuals can take proactive steps toward optimal cardiovascular health. Keep in mind to speak with your healthcare professional for precise, situation-specific advice and guidance. Embrace a heart-healthy lifestyle and empower yourself to make positive changes for your well-being and the prevention of heart failure.

Regular Checkups and Monitoring

Regular checkups and monitoring are crucial components of managing congestive heart failure (CHF) effectively.

These appointments help healthcare providers assess the progression of the condition, make necessary adjustments to the treatment plan, and monitor overall heart health. Let's delve into the comprehensive and detailed aspects of regular checkups and monitoring for CHF:

1. Frequency of Checkups:

- The frequency of checkups may vary depending on the severity and stability of your condition. Initially, more frequent appointments may be necessary, followed by regular follow-ups as recommended by your healthcare provider.

- Typically, individuals with CHF are advised to have checkups every three to six months. However, your healthcare provider will determine the appropriate schedule based on your specific needs.

2. Medical History Review:

- During each checkup, your healthcare provider will review your medical history, including previous test results, medications, symptoms, and any recent changes in your health.

- Be prepared to provide information about any new symptoms, changes in exercise tolerance, medication adherence, or lifestyle modifications you have made since your last visit.

3. Physical Examination:

- Your healthcare provider will perform a thorough physical examination, including checking your blood pressure, heart rate, breathing, and listening to your heart and lungs with a stethoscope.

- They may also examine your extremities for signs of swelling or edema.

4. Symptom Assessment:

- Your healthcare provider will assess the presence and severity of CHF symptoms, such as shortness of breath, fatigue, swelling, or rapid weight gain.

- It is important to communicate any new or worsening symptoms you have experienced since your last visit, as this information helps guide treatment decisions.

5. Medication Evaluation:

- Your healthcare provider will review your current medication regimen, assessing the effectiveness and potential side effects.

- They may make adjustments to your medications, dosages, or add new medications if necessary.

- Be sure to inform your healthcare provider about any over-the-counter medications, supplements, or herbal remedies you are taking, as they may interact with your prescribed medications.

6. Diagnostic Tests and Imaging:

- Depending on your condition and the information needed, your healthcare provider may order various diagnostic tests and imaging studies, such as echocardiograms, electrocardiograms (ECGs), stress tests, or blood tests.

- These tests provide valuable insights into your heart function, identify any changes, and help monitor the effectiveness of the treatment plan.

7. Fluid Status Assessment:

- Your healthcare provider may monitor your fluid status through methods such as regular weight checks, assessing the presence of edema, or reviewing your fluid intake and output.

- Monitoring fluid status is important for managing fluid retention and adjusting diuretic medications if needed.

8. Blood Tests:

- Blood tests, including electrolyte levels, kidney function tests, and markers of heart function (e.g., brain natriuretic peptide or BNP), may be performed to assess your overall health and the impact of CHF on your organs.

9. Lifestyle Guidance and Education:

- Regular checkups provide an opportunity for your healthcare provider to offer lifestyle guidance, including diet recommendations, exercise modifications, stress management techniques, and smoking cessation support.

- They can also provide educational resources and address any questions or concerns you may have about your condition or treatment plan.

10. Collaboration and Shared Decision-Making:

- Regular checkups foster open communication and collaboration between you and your healthcare provider. Engage in discussions, ask questions, and actively participate in shared decision-making regarding your treatment plan.

- Work with your healthcare team to set realistic goals, establish self-management strategies, and address any challenges you may encounter.

Regular checkups and monitoring are vital in managing congestive heart failure effectively. By attending these appointments, you can proactively address any changes in your condition, optimize your treatment plan, and receive ongoing support and guidance for maintaining optimal heart health. Remember to communicate openly with your healthcare provider, adhere to recommended lifestyle modifications, and follow your treatment plan to achieve the best outcomes in managing CHF.

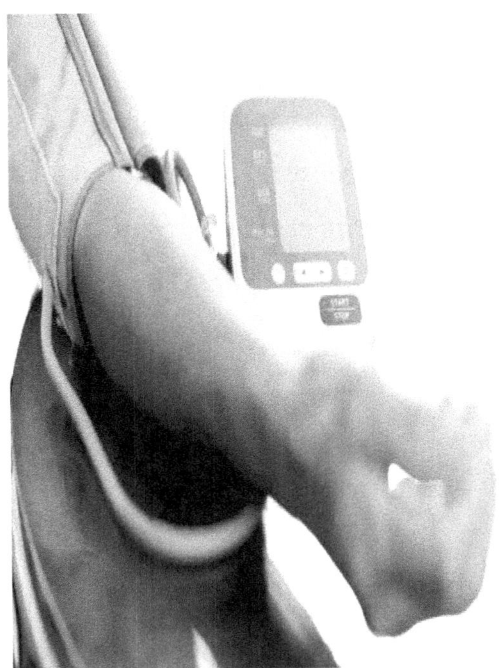

CONCLUSION

In conclusion, congestive heart failure (CHF) is a complex and potentially serious condition that requires comprehensive management and ongoing care. It occurs when the heart's ability to pump blood efficiently is compromised, leading to a range of symptoms and complications. Early detection and timely treatment are crucial in improving outcomes and enhancing quality of life for individuals with CHF.

By understanding the causes, risk factors, and early symptoms of CHF, individuals can seek prompt medical attention and begin appropriate interventions. Diagnosis involves a thorough evaluation of medical history, physical examination, and various diagnostic tests and procedures to assess heart function and identify underlying causes.

Treatment approaches for CHF encompass medications, lifestyle modifications, and, in some cases, advanced therapies or devices. Medications aim to alleviate symptoms, improve heart function, and manage underlying conditions.

Lifestyle modifications involve dietary changes, exercise, fluid restriction, and self-care practices to promote heart health and overall well-being.

Regular checkups and monitoring are essential in managing CHF effectively, allowing healthcare providers to assess the condition, adjust treatment plans, and provide ongoing support. It is important for individuals with CHF to actively participate in their care, adhere to recommended lifestyle modifications, and collaborate with their healthcare team.

While CHF poses challenges, with appropriate management and support, individuals with this condition can lead fulfilling lives. By staying informed, following medical advice, and prioritizing heart-healthy habits, individuals can optimize their heart health, manage symptoms, and improve their overall quality of life.